WHIRLWIND

To the
Shankers
with kindest
regards,

W. Francki

London 2010

WHIRLWIND

The Life & Times of a Hungarian Doctor in
the Twentieth Century

Zoltán Frankl

London & San Francisco

First published in 1995 by

The author
Dr Zoltán Frankl
85 Greenhill
Hampstead
GB-London NW3 5TZ

and also in
California:
Andrew Frankl
c/o S. Lewis
25-1 Beach Road
USA-Belvedere CA 94920

Library of Congress Cataloguing-in publication data
Whirlwind: by Zoltán Frankl

ISBN 0 952585 40 5

Manufactured in Britain

Printed by Quacks Printers, Petergate, York YO1 2HT

TO ANUCI

Contents

NOTE: All persons appearing in this book are not imaginary characters but they are all real people, and in this Autobiography not one word differs from the truth. - De mortibus nisi nihil "verum". (Of the dead nothing but the truth.)

Acknowledgements

I am very indebted to and I would like to thank Piers Plowright, Pincus and Julia Jaspert, my son Andrew Frankl, my daughter Vera and my son-in-law Etienne Duval for their encouragement, untiring effort and devotion without which this book could have never been published. There are no proper and suitable words to express my gratitude.

FOREWORD

I first met Zoltan Frankl in 1990 when a colleague and I made a BBC Radio Programme about his experiences as a Jewish oral surgeon in Mauthausen Concentration camp during the Second World War. Someone had sent me the manuscript which forms the basis of this book and I was immediately impressed by his dispassionate yet moving account of endurance under terrible conditions.

Zoltan Frankl is not a political man, nor is he interested in power. His guiding motto has always been the Latin tag "Nil Nocere" - "Harm Nothing" and his life in and outside Hungary has been dedicated to relieving human suffering. In this short account of that life, which is shot through with delightful humour as well as harrowing adventure, you will find one of the best arguments I know for being human.

Piers Plowright
January 1995

CHAPTER ONE

Childhood and Cold Water

I was born in 1907 in Kiskunhalas, Hungary. My father came from a very poor family. His father was a maker of small caps and helped round the synagogue yard. They lived in a warm, industrious, quiet Jewish home. Besides his hard work, Grandfather's main and unalterable fundamental principle was justice and honesty, he brought up his children, among them my father, in the spirit of this honesty, and this was the only heritage bequeathed to us. Grandmother died early, of tuberculosis, at the age of thirty-six, as did so many others in that dusty, neglected town of the great Hungarian Plain.

My father graduated as a doctor in 1906. It was a hard period and later he used to tell how he had walked up and down outside restaurants and satisfied himself with the smell of meals filtering out.

He was a doctor in the true sense of the word, competent in everything and an excellent physician - I still cherish his wooden stethoscope - he assisted in deliveries and treated patients with pneumonia and scarlet fever etc, but later switched to dentistry as he had to earn money to keep his family and to bring up his children. He worked with a wonderful, almost exaggerated precision, and regularly attended lectures at the Stomatological (Dental) Clinic of the University in Budapest, delivered lectures himself, and wrote scientific articles.

Mother came from Budapest. Her father mainly gambled on the Exchange so that sometimes the family had a lot of money, sometimes their furniture was taken away in a cart. Father saved her from this chaotic atmosphere and brought her into our peaceful home in Halas. She brought tenderness, goodness and love, self-sacrifice and modesty with her.

We were three brothers: Zolti, Jozsi, Sanyi - all clever, all industrious and all very naughty. We were always quarrelling and, unfortunately, that lack of understanding has run like red thread through our lives.

I have an image of Grandfather leaving our house in Halas with Father at his heels, in 1914. He was a short man in a brown suit with a brown beard and kept saying angrily that he was never going to bring us any more toys! He had come from the market and brought us a two-horse carriage made of wood. We three children began fighting over it and broke it in an instant. I never saw him again. I only remember Father running unusually fast towards the synagogue near where grandfather had lived. I can still see him in his hat and long overcoat. Mother and we three boys followed the hearse in a carriage, Father on foot, with a handkerchief in his hand. It was then I saw him crying for the first time. I was seven years old, I had not met death before and on the way back from the cemetery I was acting the clown and making childish jokes. Mother, for the first and last time in my life slapped my face. I began crying, and Father's sister Fanny remarked "He is surely crying because he is in mourning for Grandfather".

Our house at 25, later 27, Kossuth Street was L-shaped. In the shorter wing, which looked out onto the street, there was the waiting room and surgery. In the longer wing, beginning with windows looking onto the street, there was the dining room, the guest room, my parents' bedroom, the nursery, the bathroom, a small corridor next to the modern lavatory. This was followed by a large kitchen, pantry and the domestic's room. Next to the loft staircase there was an empty space for the calendar and behind it another room for the tools. Then came the stable, and next to it the back house cesspit with wooden seats over it, with a big hole for Father, and two lower and smaller ones for me and Jozsi, and finally, a tin chamber pot for Sanyi. The pit was several metres deep.

From time to time the gypsies emptied it and all the windows had to be closed for a considerable time. My favourite pastime was letting myself down and hoisting myself up through Father's great hole, balancing on my hands, never worried that I might fall into it!

Behind the house we had about half an acre of garden. Nearest the house was a small flower garden with two lilac shrubs planted by my grandfather, and a well. We fetched drinking water in large cans from the artesian well round the corner. In the garden there was a four-metre high, cone-shaped hen house. The vegetable garden was full of lettuce, string beans, tomatoes, potatoes ... and apple trees. We also had a quince tree, and its fruit was always ripe by the Day of Atonement. We stuck a clove into it to take to the synagogue to smell during fasting. We had fun climbing trees and fishing objects from the branches with pieces of string. At the end of the garden we dug a track for shot-putting. Jozsi was always the winner of these contests. Finally, we had a bower, a small wooden summerhouse overgrown with wild vine where, in fine weather, we always had our meals.

One morning, Mother ran sobbing from the kitchen towards the surgery with a telegram in her hand. Her father had died. They travelled to the funeral together. I remember sitting on this grandfather's lap, playing with his gold watch chain, in his flat in Budapest. Mother was good, patient and loving but her family exploited her wickedly and treated her almost like a stepchild. Unfortunately, so did we.

Mother's mother died when she was old and senile, in Joseph Boulevard, Budapest. I can still remember the particular smell of their staircase, and can hear the constant noise of rattling, ringing trams as I tried to sleep in their flat.

Father was a 'pater familias' in the true sense of the word! He had a passionate love for his family, but he did not tolerate any questioning of his authority. When we were 6-7 years old we still had to go to bed at 6 p.m. He expected us to be excellent pupils and when once, for the first and last time in my life I brought a bad mark home, I got such a box on my ears that it made my head swim. He was proud of us and wanted us to excel in everything. At school celebrations I always had to be among those reciting a poem. I learned to play the violin from Mrs Babo, a pupil of the famous Hungarian violinist and composer Jeno Hubay (1858-1937). Father paid a 10-crown gold coin for each lesson. The main emphasis was on my little finger being on the bow. I practised four hours a day in the garden, and finally I got as far as the Mendelssohn violin concerto. But alas, I had no real ear for music. I was a member of the students' orchestra and of the so-called 'gentry orchestra'. Once, when the latter was rehearsing, our conductor, Professor Bertalan, gave the orchestra a signal with his baton to stop, and pointing to where I was sitting said "Someone there is playing out of tune". After that I always moved the bow well above the strings, thinking it would not be noticed if one violin did not sound.

The emphasis was always on learning, from primary school through grammar school to my last examination at the University. At the Jewish Primary school the best pupil sat in the first row on the right; I should have sat there but Koralek took my place because he was the nephew of Mr Schwartz, our teacher of religion. This was the first disappointment in the course of my school years. When I had finished University, due to my excellent results all along my studies, I expected to be inaugurated 'sub-auspiciis gubernatoris', that is, I would be awarded the ring of the governor. However, Professor Bela Entz, a family friend, called me and said "Zolti, don't wait for the governor's ring any longer, you are a Jew and therefore you will never get it".

Our parents took immense care of our education. Even when we were primary school children, a German governess was brought from Stuttgart, who took us to, and fetched us from, school, and spoke German to us. We three boys were brought up extremely rigorously, hermetically even, and we had not the vaguest idea, for example, what a naked woman looked like. Thus it happened that once, when the governess was lying ill in her small room - I went in to her and slowly began slipping my hand under her eiderdown to see what she was made of. When she looked at me with a weary, indulgent smile, then, equally quietly, I withdrew my hand. I remember there was something nice, gentle, and chivalrous in this act. Once, when we were fed up with her, we pulled the chair from under her and, holding a dish of tomato juice in her hands, she fell back flat. Next day she left.

Later we had a very pretty chambermaid. One night I went into her room, silently. Nothing happened. I was very inexperienced. When I returned to my bed I was surprised to see an extra blanket on it. Mother had put it there so that her little Zolti should not catch a cold. The event was never brought up afterwards.

There was only one activity that stopped my brothers and me from quarrelling, stamp-collecting. We founded a company under the name of *Frankl Brothers* and we did business and exchanged stamps with many foreign countries. The love of stamps lasted for decades. I was already a respectable doctor when in Budapest, while having our afternoon tea, a valuable stamp slipped out of my tweezers and fell into my hot cup of tea, and this immediately dissolved part of the gum coating. I have never forgotten the shock I had then. When my son Andris left Hungary after the Revolution, I gave him my beautiful old Austrian series so that he should not be without money in Vienna. Every State values its own stamps highest. Naturally, he was cheated and hardly received anything for them.

Mother prepared the religious holidays marvellously. Pesach-Passover evenings were unforgettable - Father, leading the prayers. Orthodoxy filled our souls. We were distressed when by chance we found a farthing in our pockets on the Day of Atonement and we hastened to get rid of it. We could read Hebrew as we could read Hungarian, and we looked with devotion at the cardboard model of King Solomon's destroyed Temple which Uncle Schwartz showed to the class as a reward. Later, Uncle Schwartz was destroyed too. Mother used to sit separately in the gallery of the synagogue reserved for women. The air was stuffy and suffocating up there and sometimes she dragged herself down, or we had to carry her down. This cooled my religious enthusiasm a little. And then we were different from the majority of the other citizens. Father believed in assimilation. He was anti-Zionist and was convinced that we could merge into the community honestly, decently and without having to give up our self-respect. About this, as about so many other things, his opinion was "Excel yourself, but never become conspicuous".

We had a cow called Cifra, and in the cowshed we stored hay up in the loft. Cifra was a yellowish-brown kind of animal and we were very fond of her - maybe she was fond of us too, but once when I approached her with a large pail to milk her, she struck me in the face with her mucky tail so that I immediately gave up this 'entertainment'. The cow had a small calf and we used to jump about with it in the yard.

Then we had a little dog called Bodri that could wag its tail sweetly; the only trouble was that once it pulled off the skirt of a female patient who had hardly entered the house. Father got rid of the dog the following day. We also had nine cats: Ciru, Mici, Misi, Ilus, Cuncurka, Inci, Minci, Pinci, Cinci. Mother used to call Cuncurka 'Redhead'. They were lovely cats and when I called to them they ran home from the neighbourhood, from the roof, or wherever they were, and queued up, on their hind legs, asking for their huge meals. In spring the caterwauling at night was rather disturbing and we could not get used to it, but we could pull our blankets over our heads.

At about the same time as Bodri disappeared so did one of our chambermaids. She had taken us for a walk to the railway station where a young soldier had just been crushed to death between the buffers of two railway carriages. The poor young man had a very yellow, unreal face, and this was what she made us look at, at considerable length. My parents were not best pleased when we gave them a detailed report of the accident.

On the other hand, it was Father who showed me my first dead body. She was his uncle's wife who, according to Jewish tradition, was lying on the floor, her face yellow as wax. The mirrors were covered with white sheets.

We children slept in our own room. There was one separate bed crosswise for me and two lengthwise next to each other for Jozsi and Sanyi. There we played, clowned and giggled together. We were protected, we had no problems apart from learning and that we liked doing. There was also a small iron stove in the room. I remember well I used to sit by it with my mother, who taught me the letters of the alphabet in front of the glowing embers.

A strolling company arrived at the theatre in Halas, and it was then that I fell in love for the first time in my life. She was a slim little blondish-brown chorus girl, or perhaps it was the 'daughter' of a chorus girl. We were both fourteen and it was great, sitting in the dark auditorium gently holding hands. When they left Halas the whole class thronged to the window on the first floor of the gymnasium to see my 'love' passing.

Later, I must have been sixteen or seventeen when I went to see my mother's brother, Uncle Joska. We were talking about women's affairs - a pretty girl with a wonderful figure was with him in the surgery. Suddenly he said he had to leave us for a short time. I was left alone with the girl and I did not know what to do. In the corner I caught sight of a 10 Kg dumb-bell and I told the girl to watch me. I lifted the weight up 35 times and regarded her with proud triumph. Then Joska came back and asked what we had been doing. He couldn't believe his ears, and began kissing the girl who nestled close to him happily. I too, began stroking the girl, but by then I was 'dumb-belled'. Anyway, I asked Joska whether one has to use a condom in similar cases, and his answer was affirmative.

At my final examination at the secondary school I had to translate a text by Tacitus, the most difficult of Latin historians. My teacher came up to me and asked if I knew every word. I thanked him and said I did not need any help, I knew everything. In Hungarian literature, the poet Janos Vajda (1827-1897) was my favourite. I studied him for my thesis and knew twenty-four of his poems off by heart. I started to recite his first poem 'Forest-fire'. In a few minutes I was stopped, for they saw the enormous amount I knew. To this day, it hurts me that they did not let me recite everything.

Whilst in the fifth or sixth grade at grammar school I had a fight with a classmate called Antal Kocsis, who finally punched me in the face. To my shame I dared not hit him back and my cowardice has hurt me ever since. Yet fate willed it that Antal Kocsis became a doctor as well and it was he who anaesthetized my mother with such affection when Dr M. operated on her abscess around her kidney. So perhaps it was for the best that I had not continued fighting then - anyway I would probably have been beaten.

Our teacher of physical education was Sandor Nagykalozi. He was a convinced anti-Semite but he appreciated good performances. When at a gymnastics competition I had made the so-called 'Great Death Circle' on the horizontal bar, he said to the boys standing around "Look what one can perform with will and endurance. With his well-developed muscles he has lifted his big buttocks through the bar without touching it" - and I did win the medal. Nagykalozi had a slogan by which he encouraged members of the class to wash: *"The water isn't cold, it is only the decision to use it that is difficult"*. I have never forgotten this.

We had the traditional banquet after the final examination, at the nearby 'Salt-Lake Baths', and when it was over I went down to the lake shore with some of my companions. As we stood by the smooth water of the silent lake I looked in vain for some sign. What would happen to all of us - no longer students, not yet men? No answer from the water.

CHAPTER TWO

Lecturers, Lechery and Love

(1925-1931)

We Jewish young men admitted to the University of Pecs formed a close-knit group. My elder brother, Jozsi, and four other students, being a year younger than me, attended the course below me. I was the sixth to join their group so we assumed the name 'The Six'. We kept together in everything. We played billiards together in a café, we went to parties, out with girls, and on excursions together. We also played cards together, but mainly we studied.

'R', our lecturer in physics, was a grey, simple, straightforward man. You had to learn his book and then you could pass the examination successfully. The chemistry lectures of Z. were much more interesting with many colourful experiments. Once he showed us a substance in the form of a white powder in a small vial, and said this was responsible for the abominably foul smell of country cesspools. The substance was called *Scatol*, from its chemical name *beta-methyl-indol*. My friend Zoltán Darvas and myself named it 'crystalline muck' and we were wondering into whose pocket we could put a speck of it; whoever it was could never have used his suit again.

The Professor of Anatomy was T.Zs., formerly chief medical officer somewhere. He was a notorious anti-Semite, an ignorant man with a perverse habit of tugging away at his moustache. He delivered lectures on anthropology as well and, if you wanted to pass the examination, you had to participate in those lectures.

T.Zs liked to illustrate his lectures with his own coloured drawings. He hated Jews but appreciated my knowledge and once, when a problem arose about the accuracy of a figure, he called me into his room to ask my opinion, which was practically unimaginable then.

It is characteristic of our preparation for anatomy that we bought a brain, wrapped it up carefully, took it home and, placing it on our table, studied long into the nights the complicated convolutions. Naturally we took it back to the Institute, for the funeral.

Stout Uncle G. was a kind, wise man. From him we gathered the basic principles of biology; we stimulated the nerves of frogs' legs with electric current and observed the muscular contractions. I really made use of my knowledge of Greek at these lectures - I only wish I had learned English as well.

I learned paediatrics from another notorious anti-Semite H. and sat my examination under him. My paper was identical to the paper of S., a Christian. He received the mark *Excellent*; I received the mark *Good*. This injustice made me so indignant that I asked to be given a hearing: how was it possible to mark two identical papers differently? He accepted my argument but asked me in turn what could be done now, as he had already written *Good* into my lecture book. Observing my silence and realizing that he had been unjust, he finally said he would write 'Very' before the word Good, that Very Good meant always Excellent.

R.C. was Professor of Psychology and was at least as psychopathic as his patients. His examinations were notorious. I spent my internship in his department, and one morning met an elderly patient, Mr. Kohn, in a ward, suffering from senile mental disturbance. The characteristic feature of this disease is that the patient's brain does not perceive recent things, but only remembers old events, those of his childhood. Knowing this, I started to pray in Hebrew: "Nismasz kol haj tvoreh es szimcho Adonaj elauhenu". ("The soul of every living being shall bless thy name, O Lord our

God.") He looked at me intently and continued smoothly: "Vruah kol boszor tfoer uszraumem zichrochu malkenu.." ("And the spirit of flesh shall glorify and exalt thy memorial, O our King..") Then I began the Passover Prayer: "Avodim hojinu lfaraj bmicrajim.." ("We were slaves to Pharaoh in Egypt.."), whereupon he: "bjod hazoko uvizraja ntujo.."("With strong hands and outstretched hands ..") Then, his eyes sparkling, he sang with me: "Had gadjo, had gadjo dizvan abo biszre zuze had gadjo .." ("An only kid, an only one which my father bought for two zuzim, an only kid..") Then I told the grace before eating bread: "Boruch atto Adonaj elauhenu meleh hoalom hamauci lechem min hoorec .." ("Blessed art thou, O Lord our God, King of the Universe, who bringest forth bread from the earth..")

He looked at me with sparkling eyes, he was infinitely happy. His thinking, his soul being at home in his country, his brain was functioning flawlessly. Then he asked me: "Are you a Bocher?" ("Young religious teacher".)

I could not answer for R. was coming on one of his rounds with his entourage, and I disappeared like a flash of lightning. R. went to Mr. Kohn first and asked him how he was and he, as if waking from a doze, pointed around and said: "This man knows everything." R. went to the next patient unimpressed. Only I knew what these words meant, and was pleased I was able to make a fellow human really happy for ten or fifteen minutes. I spent only a month at the mental hospital, but even this short time had such an effect on me that, when I finished my activities there, I could hardly adapt myself to the outside world. I thought that that was the real world.

I have another unforgettable memory of that Institute. Every morning on my arrival, I would find a thirty to thirty-five year old woman simply but properly dressed, with a normal face and intelligent eyes, standing at a first floor window with a bundle in front of her on the window sill. Her hands were on the bundle as she looked motionlessly out onto the courtyard. I started talking to her and asked her what she was doing; her answer was always the same: "I am expecting to be fetched and taken home." Two years later, my brother Sanyi went to the hospital to serve his internship. The woman was still standing at the window and raised her eyes to my brother and asked simply: "Have you come back again, Dr Frankl?" Sanyi, who looked very much like me, had the surprise of his life, and I too was deeply moved when he told me what had happen. There are many things which are not within our knowledge.

Professor Entz's lectures on pathology were splendid. He mixed otherwise dry and difficult topics with such profound humour that everything seemed to be easy and simple. On one occasion he presented a cardiac death caused by a stabbing (quite a frequent occurrence in those days) but, in addition to the pathological description, he gave a detailed description of the drunken brawl that might have led up to the fatality. A group of lads coming out of a pub had started fighting over some disagreement about a girl; then one of the lads, a hothead, suddenly whipping out a jack-knife from his boot stabbed one of his drinking partners in the back! The knife penetrated the heart, and soon led to cardiac arrest. No-one could ever forget this pathological case report. My respected and beloved colleague, Zoltán Darvas, who was among the students, burst into paroxysms of uncontrollable laughter when Entz demonstrated whipping the jack-knife out of the boot, so much so that the lecture nearly had to be interrupted. Entz was visibly very pleased. His book called *Small-size Entz*, was our bible and, even now, after sixty years, I often take it out of my bookcase.

His teaching was always interwoven with humour and, as a family friend, he sometimes made personal allusions. His demonstrations were immortal. The audience were either sitting or standing on one side of the dissecting table and the Professor was taking around different organs on a large tray and asking everyone a question on the material calling everybody by their name. On one occasion he asked one of my brothers: "Mr Sandor Frankl, what do you see?" Sanyi did not see anything. I was standing by the dissecting table in my white gown, for I used to visit the Institute, and Professor Entz, walking round the semicircle came back behind the table. He turned to me and asked me if I saw anything. "The kidney is penetrated by pus", was my answer. "You see, he sees it", cried the Professor triumphantly, and continued to say that there was going to be a great scandal and great sorrow at dinner time in Siklosi Street, for Zoltán Frankl had recognized what Sandor did not.

In 1930 I spent three months at a sanatorium in Davos on account of an initial bleeding from the lung and when at my examination in Forensic Medicine I had to speak about the organs of the chest, he had the chest opened by the attendant, so as not to overstrain me. Twenty years later, when in the great lecture hall of the Surgical Department of the University of Pecs, I reported on my clinical and anatomical investigations concerning the area around the throat, he was sitting in the front row, arms crossed, grey moustache, short greyish hair standing upright, and not taking his eyes off me for a moment. I think he was the only one who really understood my rather complicated and lengthy discussions. After the lecture, he came up to me and told me my Father would be very proud of me if he were able to be here now. Later, he wrote to me that it was quite incredible to produce anything new in such an ancient and so well-known field of anatomy, but with zeal and will I had done so.

If possible, I always sent my material requiring pathological investigation down to him from Budapest, and could always, always learn from him, his wise findings extending to the smallest details. At the exposure of the left side of the lower jaw, I found in one of my patients a progressive tissue proliferation that could not be identified with anything. It extended to such depth that I could not follow it to the end. I sent the removed tissues to an Associate Professor of Pathology in Budapest who diagnosed it to be a malignant tumour. The patient was an opera singer and radical surgery - the total removal of his left lower jaw - would have meant the end of his career. I do not remember any more how, but I had kept some of the removed tissue specimens, which I immediately sent to Pecs, to Professor Entz. In three days I received the answer by telegram: "The histology does not show any malignancy, no need for radical intervention". My patient continued singing happily for many years.

In addition to pathology, Entz was also Professor of Forensic Medicine. After his retirement he dealt with archaeological research of the Avar Tombs excavated in the surroundings of Pecs. He was particularly concerned with the examination of teeth. He said then that he never would have thought that teeth could play such an important rôle in archaeological investigations.

He always emphasized he did not want to teach us rare case histories which we would probably never meet in our practice, but rather everyday diseases such as pneumonia. It was his teachings that remained longest in our memories.

He was a charming, cheerful, good-humoured man. During many years I only saw him once lose his composure, when he had to perform the autopsy of a twenty-two year old student of his who had died from pulmonary tuberculosis. Then, he put down his scalpel and earnestly and very sadly said "Life is shit!"

We learned internal medicine from A. who was a very decent, honest man, but he spoke extremely slowly and his lectures were immeasurably boring and he spoke about typhoid fever for at least a whole term. On the other hand, our lecturer on medical diagnostics was R. and his teaching was really suited for general practitioners. We liked him very much. I got into personal contact with him when, in our room in Siklosi Street, I had a sudden pulmonary haemorrhage. Rutich was not allowed to see private patients but he was the

15

only one I had confidence in. Jozsi could not do anything else but keep pressing his head on my chest to stop the bleeding. All the same, my brothers succeeded in persuading Rutich to come and see one of his students, and he did come. I asked him two questions: "Am I going to bleed to death?" and: "Am I going to asphyxiate from bleeding?" He reassured me and had me taken to the Pulmonary Unit of A's Clinic.

This type of bleeding is in the initial form of tuberculosis, a warning, so to say. I was not critically ill and, after the first scare, I soon recovered. Meanwhile, I began helping in the laboratory. I was greatly distressed that I could not continue my studies; however, I had become resigned to it. Sometimes I felt like singing, and I began to sing my favourite Hungarian folk songs. The singing became louder and louder and I drummed the rhythm on my bedside table. My roommates soon joined in and then patients from other wards, what's more, nurses and laboratory workers all joined in until a stentorian voice warned: "The Doctors are coming". Everything became silent and we lay in our beds like severely ill patients.

I spent three months at A's Clinic, then Father sent me to Davos for a further three months. In Davos I stayed at Dr B.'s Sanatorium. He was of Hungarian origin and, because I was a doctor's son and a medical student myself, gave me 'preferential' treatment. In my case he did not accommodate me in the main building but in another wooden storeyed annex. My treatment consisted of my temperature being taken regularly, and lying on the balcony for two or three hours mornings and afternoons, breathing in the crystal-pure Swiss air.

It was 1929, I was young and twenty-two years old, so no wonder that I felt an extreme desire for the other sex.

I used to smother the little Swiss chambermaid bringing me my breakfast, with embraces. It was a miracle that the coffee was not spilt on my bed! Then, one afternoon, being bored, I went for a walk into Davos. Unexpectedly, on the second or third floor window of a house, I noticed a woman tidying up the room, and she noticed me too. I signalled to her with my handkerchief, she waved back and then dropped a note in which she indicated our meeting place. I returned to the sanatorium where I found the following note on my bed: "During Doctor's rounds you were absent. I warn you, this should not happen again! Biro. Head Physician". Well, in the following days, we had many joyful hours on the grassy, warm slope of the hill. There was a Hungarian doctor occupying the room next to mine and I told him the story. He sighed: "Zoltán, if you could, only once, get a woman for me too". Naturally I promised to do my best. On the next occasion, I asked my partner if she had a friend for my colleague, as he was also longing for a girl. Next time, she appeared with one of her friends who first stood on guard while we were enjoying ourselves in the meadow. Then I started walking with her towards the sanatorium. I had not known what a dangerous task I had undertaken; namely that our building was not a real house built of brick, but a wooden structure, for those who paid less. The stairs creaked terribly and, as I should have been in bed hours earlier, we climbed extremely carefully in constant fear. On arriving upstairs, I opened my colleague's door and told him I had brought the promised woman. I can still see his thin face with his thick moustache when, half rising in his bed, he said, alarmed: "Oh no, not now!" Disappointed, I closed the door and seeing the crestfallen woman beside me, I took her to my room to console her. My colleague and I never spoke again about affairs with women!

My first great love in Pecs was young Bozsi R. I was full of fire and restlessness. Every Friday night we rushed to the Reformed Synagogue, running from the central building of the University so as not to be late. To greet Sabbath, the eternally young bride, as it is written. The men were sitting on the ground floor, we students standing behind them. The gallery, right and left, packed with women and girls. When they stood up, the bar covered them only up to their waist. Bozsi was there too, on the left. The eyes of all the boys found heaven in the gallery.

In quiet, as well as stormy, evenings, I used to walk below her window in the square outside the synagogue until she had turned off the light. Second floor, fourth window on the left. And I imagined her getting into her bed, under her laced quilt, slowly closing her lovely brown eyes. I even wrote a poem about her, that was published in the local paper. The price of these heroic longings was many a sore throat and hoarseness. She became someone else's wife. Anyway, I was only a medical student then, and she was courted by a professor's assistant. Twenty years later, when she already had grown-up children, I reminded her of old times, I learned from her that her window had been the first on the left, and that the fourth window belonged to a small room occupied by her old lame, hairy aunt! Naturally this trifle did not change my memories.

My other love affair was with Elly, who could say "Zolti" in such a lovely way. She was a short, very pretty girl with black hair and fiery eyes. She always sang. They had a grocery store and, when in the evening I was ambling home from the University, she used to sit in the window of the first floor doing her sewing and answered my whistling with a happy laugh.

When we were coming downhill from the Department of Obstetrics for our next lecture at the Clinic of Ophthalmology, I used to pop in for a kiss. Nothing more happened between us, and I was always a little late at the Ophthalmology lectures. One of my colleagues, Steven Flesch, was also courting Elly and my frequent journeys in that direction roused his suspicions. Once, during a lecture, a sudden restlessness caught him. He jumped up, left the lecture hall, took a tram and visited Elly. She was in bed with a cold and I was sitting at her bedside quietly holding her hand. Well, there is such a thing as telepathy. Later, Elly married a football player.

The natural outcome of our strict education at home and of the seclusion from girls and women was that hardly had we been liberated from paternal supervision and got to University at Pecs, before we threw ourselves savagely upon women. We became regular visitors of the brothels in Timor Street. The girls knew us well and awaited us eagerly and agreed without objection that "the first time" does not count, for hardly had we touched them and it was over. We always kept in mind the preventative measures Father had taught us. Once, I felt some itching and I lifted a little moving thing out of my pubic hairs. It was a louse. I looked at it under my Zeiss microscope and I saw such a huge monster with hairy feet that I nearly fainted! Then, there came the treatment; sterilisation of my clothes, etc. In short, sexual life did not always consist of sheer delight. However, you could not fight against the hormones and, when I appeared below the boys' windows with the brim of my hat turned up, which meant "Ready to act", they all lined up behind me.

One night when I had got tired of learning Obstetrics, I went to bed and soon fell into a sleep. Suddenly, in the middle of the night, my brother Sanyi woke me up, kissed me, and said: "Thank you very much Zolti". The thing seemed to be a little suspicious but I soon fell asleep again. Next morning it turned out that Sanyi, returning from his mid-term holidays, was walking along Kiraly Street when a very pretty girl called out to him from the other side of the road: "So you have come back, Zolti?" Sanyi, who looked very much like me, answered: "Yes", and they spent a very pleasant evening together. Well, you can't trust fraternal kisses either ...

The Professor of Obstetrics was a short, thick-set, hot-tempered, rude, cynical, extremely right-wing man and leader of the extreme student organisation. He was a good surgeon, but an abominably bad teacher. He wrote a textbook on operative surgery and you had to mug it up word for word, if you wanted to pass the examination. If a candidate transposed two or three words, he would stop him. The consequence of this method was that, when we had finished our studies, we had not the vaguest idea about obstetrics.

Part of our training was to assist at a delivery. Our small room and the delivery room were full of dozens of cockroaches. There, I assisted with my first delivery. The following morning I sent a postcard to my parents that, at the previous dawn, I gave birth to a healthy baby girl.

In Obstetrics I spent my period of hospital training in Budapest, at the Saint Rokus Hospital. There, I performed my first and last abortion in the same operating theatre where the world-famous Semmelweis worked.

On one occasion, when the head of the foetus had already appeared, I made a bet with the midwife as to whether it was going to be a boy or a girl. She won a bottle of beer. From that day on, during deliveries, we kept humming the verse: "The little nurse succeeds, the little doctor doesn't".

In November 1931 I graduated as a doctor but - on account of my illness - three months later than my classmates. Father and Mother came to the graduation ceremony. They sat in the front row. Professor Entz as Dean of the Faculty delivered the inaugural speech. "This is a great day", he said, "parents have come from all over the country to participate in the graduation ceremony of their sons. It is at least as much their merit as that of their children, that has achieved this." And, while he was saying these words, he kept looking at my parents. And Mother quietly, softly began to weep.

CHAPTER THREE

The Story of Anuci

On a Spring evening in 1932 my friend Laci Menczel, my elder brother, and myself went on a jaunt to visit the Engel family on the outskirts of Budapest. Mr Engel was an overseer of the Chinoin Factory. Girls and boys mingled light-heartedly. There was a tall girl amongst us with black hair, who was somehow different from all the other girls I had known so far. She was taller than the others that I had courted, even her face was not that of the movie star I had imagined for myself; in short, she was not my type.

The hours passed away, the atmosphere relaxed, and whilst in the adjoining room the greater part of the company amused themselves, we switched off the light - the door was left open - and the tall, black-haired girl with her intelligent face, lay down on the sofa, holding between her fingers the indispensable cigarette, me sitting on a chair near her head, as I started to tell her my poems. Softly, melodiously; poems which I had written to other girls and recited to this tall, black-haired girl who was not 'my type', that I wanted to kiss on the mouth. She turned her head away, quietly but resolutely - but she was not cross with me.

We caught the last tram and I got off at Lehel Square with a pretty girl whom I accompanied back to her home - but only one image stuck firmly inside me, that of the girl who was sitting in her greyish-brown trench coat and beret, in the left front corner of the tram, her hands in her pockets, her body radiating vitality; so relaxed and yet so alert, with her hair flaming out sideways from under her beret.

That was how the story of Anuci and Zolti started...

A visit to Benczur Street, Long high hall, long high dining room, tall women and men, who appear at first sight to be handsome Germans. Zolti as usual has arrived late, and is seated with his back to the window. Anuci did her best, offers him coffee and cakes, showing perhaps too much effort, but anyway this gentleman is her guest. Magda, another female guest, takes a taxi home immediately, but another guest called Bandi and Zolti are walking along the street discussing the evening, saying how pretty Magda was and how sweet Anuci was. After all, it would not have been 'proper' not to mention the hostess.

An evening at Number 15 Hold Street - Anuci has moved. To start with only a few people present who have come to play bridge. Anuci bustles in front of the carved cupboard looking for knives, forks and spoons. Throwing her head back, she flings back her waving black hair and then bends down; her deep blue, red-striped pullover is lifted up above her skirt and an inch-thick area of whitish-pink slip comes into view. With a typically womanly move, she pulls the pullover down again. Her behaviour towards Zolti seems a little bit warmer.

Zolti does not play bridge as well as he would have liked and losing leaves him angry and irritable.

But the visits become more and more frequent and the number of other visitors become less and less. Anuci and Zolti sit alone on the baroque chairs beside the big radio set. Mama, Anuci's mother, sits at the table with her back to them, playing 'patience'. Mama goes to sleep.

One day Zolti takes two of his friends with him, Pali Flesch and Arpad Bernath, to introduce them to Anuci. Actually he is eager to know their opinion. The result is unanimous. Zolti is proud and delighted.

Excursion on the Danube in Vili's (Magda's friend) motorboat. Before setting out Anuci glances at the muscular figure of Zolti in his bathing suit, and does not seem very disappointed. Zolti notices. They set out: Anuci, Magda, Vili and Zolti. Zolti, lying on his back is reading a thriller while Vili, in the middle of the Danube excitedly shouting the name of Christ, keeps pulling forcibly at a frayed piece of rope as he tries for the hundredth time to put life into the motor.

The name of the wayside inn at Vac is 'Hell'. Sunset. Walk among the sparse trees in the high grass. They lie down. The first kiss. Anuci seemed to be the more active but she denies it to this day. A large dinner on the terrace and before going to sleep, Anuci and Zolti embrace on the sofa.

Nogradveroce. Walking in the moonlight. Zolti and Vili go wild, moonstruck, they start singing and reciting even after they have gone to bed, beating and thumping excitedly on the dividing wall of the women's cabin. The air is very close and damp in the cabin.

Zolti falls in love with the Danube. Anuci teaches him rowing with much love, patience and a little nervousness. Zolti's oars touch the water a lot with the flat side of the blades. He draws his oars with strength but no rhythm even though sitting in front of him he has his teacher, Anuci, with her beautiful, slightly tanned back, swinging her muscular arms.

Frici's cabin. The walls are full of photos of film stars. Anuci and Zolti are resting on the small sofa; Anuci has on a yellow bathing costume, Zolti's is black. Anuci raises her arm with a marvellous, virginal, beautiful motion ....

The rowing boat is moving fast. Mama is sitting on the shore reading, keeping an eye on her 'children'. It begins to rain and they quickly head for the shore and pull the boat up onto the Island of Szentendre. They find some canvas for cover and slip under it; the rain gets stronger and stronger - but there is not even a kiss.

Long, very long evenings at Hold Street. By the time Mama glances back, they have already drawn apart. Zolti takes leave of Anuci around midnight.

Walks, excursions. Zolti signals from the street,. The later he is, the louder the signal and the innocent pigeons flutter up, alarmed. An answer from the fifth floor. The sound of Zolti's feet on the stairs. No need to ring the bell - the door opens automatically.

Quarrels. Anuci does not like the unpunctuality. Zolti is not sure of his feelings towards Anuci. He respects her, he has a high opinion of her, but he is still not madly in love with her. Anuci wants to educate Zolti and does it unhesitatingly.

December 1932; the opening of the surgery in Rakoczi Street. Magda has some trouble with her teeth and Anuci has accompanied her. Anuci drops in another time as well; she then complains of her heart. Zolti examines her on the new couch covered with a brick-red cover which has been bought by instalments, and this, together with the monthly payment of twenty pengo for little Joly, his assistant, caused Zolti so many worries. At night, the brightness of Rakoczi Street shines into the surgery; and in Zolti's memory it shines forever: the shadows of the bent cord of the drilling machine and the big spherical lamp.

Zolti's assistant, little Joly is so very, very good to her boss. Maybe she has fallen a little bit in love with him. The surgery moves to 44 Erzsebet Boulevard and Jolyka is sitting in the van guarding the equipment. Once, after surgery hours, they go down together to the street and have a chat on the pavement. Jolyka speaks with love and kindness about Anuci, but says that she would not make a good wife because she is much cleverer than Zolti. Later Jolyka dies in St Stephen's Hospital from pneumonia. When Zolti and Sanyi visit her, for the last time, she is already dying but still conscious and when Zolti takes hold of her hand, she looks at him with her beautiful warm eyes and - somewhat apologetically -

whispers: "Zolti". This is the first time she hasn't called him "Doctor".

Eurhythmics' performance at the Magyar Theatre. "The death of the Machine". Anuci's solo dance is not just a dance, its a passionate duel between life and death. Anuci lies motionless amidst thunderous applause.

Summer 1933. Farewell at the station. It is the first time Anuci has left him. Jealousy. Anuci writes about two landowners whom she visits and with whom she goes on outings. Later, a 'phone call from the main post office; full of happiness and laughter: "My dear Anuci, do you love me?" "I love you very much, my dear Zolti!"

Anuci comes back. Zolti takes a train to Komarom to meet her. The bridge at Komarom. Sentry box. Frontier between Hungary and Czechoslovakia. Anuci comes over by a coach and takes Zolti by surprise. Intimate, quiet walk by the Danube. Sailing home by steamer. The boat sails into the night. The wind blows cold. They take shelter under the big funnel and embrace all the way to Budapest.

January 1934. Anuci, Zolti. It is uncertain who phoned who. "Ecstasy" is running in a cinema in the Terez Boulevard. The horses are magnificent and the actress looks wonderful as she rises from the surf. During the performance Anuci and Zolti reach out for each other's hands and then kiss on the mouth.

Sailing on the Danube. Excursions to Horany. 'Rugby' with Dicky. Rowing in Tibor Weisz's 'Vera'. Three of them: Anuci, Bozsi and Zolti make an excursion from the beach house at Kemendy. At the start Bozsi drops Zolti's watch into the Danube; the watch which Zolti has treasured so much since he was thirteen. Repeatedly Zolti dives in head first and down to the bottom of the ice-cold Danube, but on the pebbled riverbed there is no trace of the watch. Bozsi does not even say "Sorry".

'Soiree' at Erzsebet Boulevard, the home of the newspaper *Est*. Zolti has asked Anuci to be the hostess. The door between the waiting room and surgery is open, borrowed rows of shining cutlery, borrowed chairs and tables. Eating and drinking bouts, intelligent voices, discussions, fairy tales, laughter. Uncle Kiss who, with his wife, are our domestic help, a gentleman-like valet with his white gloves serves the dishes with them on. He takes the guests' overcoats, picks up the crumbs from the floor, grips the partly emptied glass bottles and carries them out to the kitchen until, some hours' later, the colour of the gloves change to greyish and finally black. Success, everybody is happy, but Zolti happiest of all. Anuci is wearing a light blue dress with a delicate neckline, a blue like the sunlit Italian sky. Her face looks a little tired from the excitement but her eyes are sparkling, her hair shining, her figure tall and slender.

Zolti puts his arms around her. They stand there, heads bent together. The real Lady of the House.

Zolti's rugby playing friend Dicky visits Anuci one afternoon. They have a chat. Anuci plays with a little ring. Dicky asks her "Is it new?" Anuci replies "Yes". "Who did you get it from?" asks Dicky. Anuci, prompted by a light-hearted idea, says "From Joska Reichardt". Dicky, surprised says: "From Reichardt, not from Zolti?" Anuci replies: "Yes, really, from Reichardt, I've become engaged to him". With a deep sigh Dicky says: "Poor Zolti". He glances at her reproachfully and leaves.

Next day, Saturday morning at Zolti's flat. Anuci has already informed Zolti of what had happened. Mrs Kiss, the housekeeper, welcomes Dicky into the hall. When Dicky asks how the doctor is Mrs Kiss cries into her handkerchief: "Dear me, what will happen now to our poor Doctor?" Zolti is lying on his bed and answers Dicky's mournful greetings with scarcely audible moaning. Dicky, in black overcoat and holding a black hat, pulls a chair near to the bed. Ten or fifteen minutes pass in silence. Zolti wriggles under his blanket, pressing his fingernails hard into his own flesh, and nearly exploding from pent-up laughter. Dicky tries very hard to hold back his tears. Then came Dicky's consolation speech. "Dear Zolti, don't worry. Of course, it's impossible to forget Anuci. You will never, ever find anybody like her but, nevertheless my dear fellow, don't worry." Having said this he stands up and, with the sternness which would have put even a funeral procession to shame, he leaves. Zolti is half-dead already.

1935. Professor Adam's Clinic. Surgical operations. Before nightfall some rejoicing usually, in the Clinic. Anuci visits her boyfriend. She also brings some supplement to dinner. They go up to the dining room but Anuci eats the quail. They meet again in the Duty Room. Fervent kisses, big embraces. Anuci sets out for the gate and Zolti for the 5th Sick Ward. He looks and waves back until Anuci's shadow is hidden by the darkness of the peaceful courtyard. "Oh how good it is, we were just waiting for you dear Doctor, there are some injections prepared for you!"

'Roman' swimming pool at the Danube. Ervin's boathouse. Tiled floor and a colourful curtain, a couch with a coloured pillow. There are no bounds and limits to embracing. Anuci's eyes are glittering moistly, Zolti kisses her hand with enthusiastic devotion. They close the door carefully. They go upstairs to the Magashazy's Restaurant floor for dinner. The music blares from the riverside, in competition with the music from the gramophones on the boats; the sunset breeze brings along thousands and thousands of confessions of love, crying, laughter, dancing rhythms and screaming songs. The lamps light up slowly here and there, even the jealous sky gradually shows forth its stars.

19th December 1935. Wedding ceremony. On the previous day there have been awkward scenes with the fitting of the jacket and tie. Top hat. Rushing headlong and bursting into Hold Street, a little late. Anuci is ready. They put on the head-dress. And, as is customary, surrounded by the people who live in the house, passers-by and various onlookers, Anuci and Zolti get into the taxi which has been covered with white flowers. The 5th District Registry Office. They have to wait because another wedding ceremony is in progress. Then "Yes", given in a firm voice by both. The mothers are weeping softly into their handkerchiefs. After the official last words, a metal candlestick falls off the table onto the ground with a crash. "Mazltov!" says Professor Simon. The Synagogue in Csaky Street. Zolti and Anuci are placed in small, separate compartments on opposite sides of the Ark containing the Torah. Now they are standing under the 'hupe' - the wedding tent. The Rabbi starts the ceremony. "I have known the bride for decades" - and here he paused for rather a long time - "I have heard only beautiful and good things about the bride's family. The woman is the spirit of the Jewish hearth ..." and then, turning to Zolti, he continued in a drawling, rather sorrowful voice: "And you dear, good bridegroom ..."

Anuci and Zolti press their fingernails into their palms and do their best to preserve the dignity of the occasion. Beside the Rabbi stands a young Cantor with passionate eyes. Anuci wears a white, silk dress with an arrow-like interwoven silver thread design running from the upper edge of the dress and ending somewhere below the midriff. The Cantor does not take his eyes off her throughout the sermon.

Lunch at the Café New York in the Marble Room, in the same café where Anuci and Zolti had had so many wonderful lunches sitting comfortably on red velvet-backed chairs, surrounded by an army of familiar, kind waiters.

The lunch is excellent, the table settings splendid, the aroma of the delicate dishes ... everything is a great success. Only on the fork of the newly-wed young woman an incriminating remnant of spinach from the previous day. Anuci, as ever, the 'mistress' of the situation as she hands the fork over to her old friend, the Head Waiter ... who hangs it in the kitchen, attached to a string; a fork with a piece of spinach stuck to it - an ironic memento of the wedding lunch.

They go home. Some patients were waiting for Zolti and he works until evening. Anuci meanwhile sits on the dustbin in her kitchen, in her white wedding dress ... Later, Anuci sleeps on Zolti's bed couch with Zolti next to her on a mattress on the floor. Next day they depart. Through snow drifts, in a 2nd class Pullman carriage to Vienna. By taxi to the Imperial. Too expensive. So they ask the driver to take them to another good, but not so expensive, place - the Hotel Windsor.

They are still in bed in the morning when someone knocks on the door. It is Robert, Anuci's Uncle. Leaning against the bed he asks how they got there. They told him and he roars with laughter. The Windsor Hotel, he tells them, is widely known as a 'flop-house'. It does not matter. It gives an extra piquancy to their kisses. However, there is no way of getting a clothes brush in the 'Hotel'. Perhaps it hasn't been needed very much before.

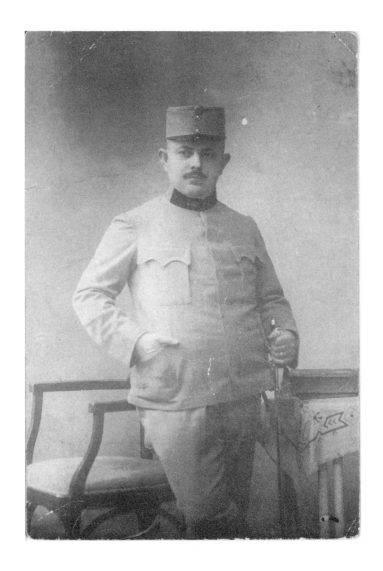

*The author's father, a medical officer in the
Austro-Hungarian Army, 1915*

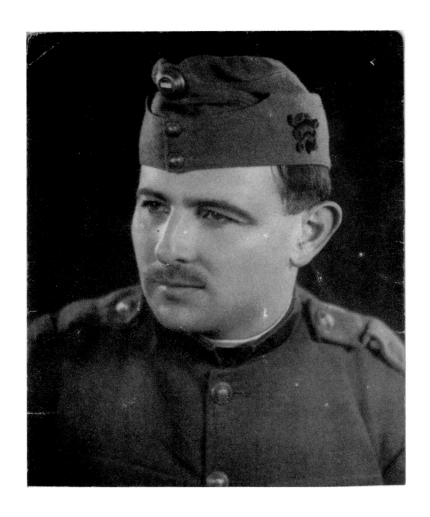

*Zoltán Frankl as a Private in the Army
of the Hungarian Republic, 1939*

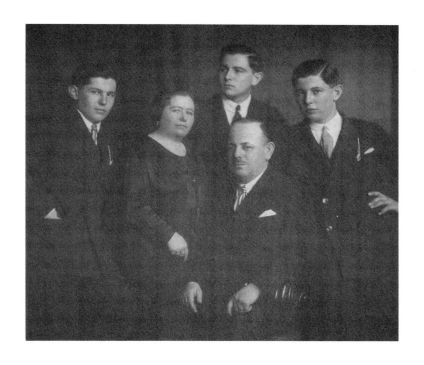

A family group in 1924: Jozsef, the author's mother, with her son - the author - and husband, and Sandor

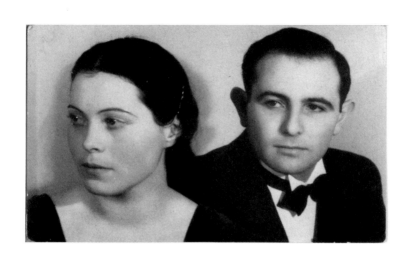

The wedding in 1935: Anuci (Anna) and Zoltán Frankl

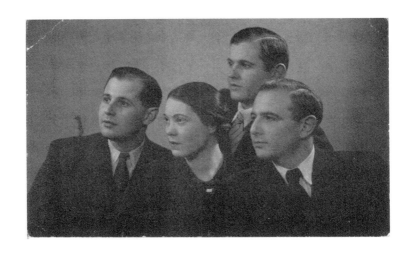

*A family group in 1936: Sandor, Anuci, Jozsef
and the author*

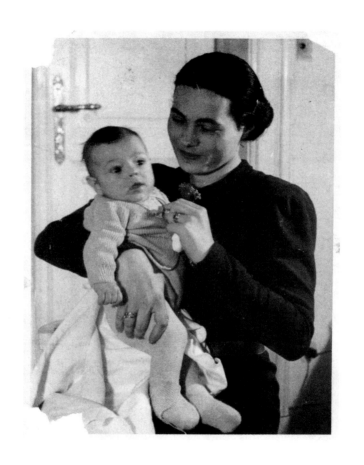

Anuci with Baby Andris in 1938

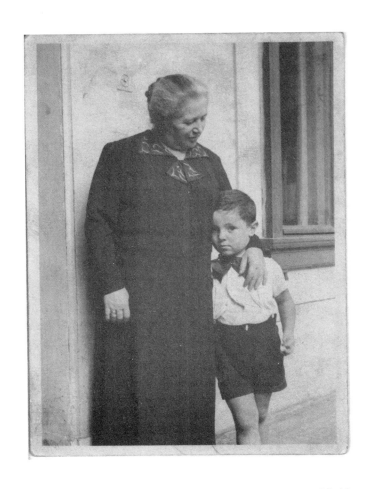

The author's mother with her grandson in 1941

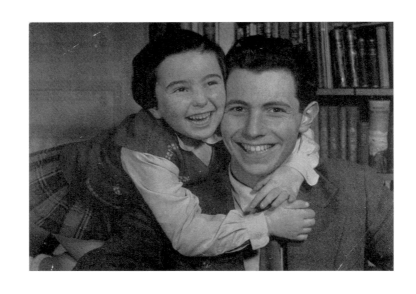

*Vera and Andris before leaving Hungary
in the spring of 1956*

CHAPTER FOUR

Labour - Free & Forced

(1931-1940)

I was a second-year medical student when Father arranged with Dr M., Chief of the Hospital on the outskirts of Kiskunhalas, that I could go to the Hospital as an observer. M. was an excellent surgeon; he had come from one of the surgical clinics in Budapest to organise and work. He worked beautifully and successfully. I snooped about, peeping here and there, trying to get the atmosphere of the Hospital and mainly got the smell of ether! I stained blood cells in the small laboratory, peeped in at autopsies, and watched surgical interventions, the mysteries of scrubbing, giving injections, and putting on sterile gowns. One day, there was a hernia operation. The patient was a well-built, strong young man - an agricultural worker. The operation was a simple unilateral hernia of the groin, one of the first surgical interventions young surgeons are allowed to perform. Everything went smoothly and the patient was put into a four-bed ward, the first bed on the left. The following morning, I went to see how he was and found his bed empty. Earlier on, they had tried to awaken him but he was dead; a blood clot in the artery of the lung. At the post mortem there it was, riding dark and red. I was very sad but learned then, and never forgot, that there is no such thing as a 'minor' operation.

During my university years, I never knew what branch of medicine I wanted to specialise in. What I did know, and insisted upon, was that, under no circumstances did I want anything to do with dental surgery; I was a physician through and through, or so I thought. But fate dictated otherwise and, of all places, in the men's toilets at the Stomatological Clinic.

My dear father regularly took part in scientific sessions there and by chance happened to be in the said toilets with Professor Szabo - the Director of the Clinic. My father turned to Szabo and said "Dear Professor, please take my son into your clinic, he has passed all his studies from beginning to end, with distinction". Szabo replied: "Of course, Aron, just send him along". That was it. The matter of my future was decided there and then. Being Jewish, it would have been difficult to get into any other clinic and, in any event, my parents secretly wanted me to take over the dental practice in Kiskunhalas. It all happened after I had just graduated, I was tired, apathetic and in no position to oppose it. So be it.

My entry was not enthusiastically received as the course had started 2½ months before and, to catch up I had to have and pay for, extra tuition from two assistant professors. At first I worked in the laboratory carving teeth from oblong pieces of wax, teeth which resembled more the clubs of a fighting prehistoric man!

Assistant Professor Sz. taught 'local anaesthesia' in one small room and, in the larger room next door, we performed the extractions. My record was 35 in one hour. The removal of roots which were pushed to the cavity of the upper jaw were left to my elder colleague, an excellent man who was to leave us for Israel. In the Conservative Department my first teacher was Dr E. Balazs, a charming man who, with his wife, joined our circle of friends. He mentioned to his wife one evening that a new, talented student, somewhat strong headed, had joined him and nearly injured the mouth of one of his patients with a paper disc. His wife enquired "Was it Zolti Frankl, by any chance?"

The year went slowly by and I passed the examination. I remember the porter, (Uncle Mihaly), at the Clinic, who would turn a blind eye when I used to phone Anuci and when, in 1956, my son Andris was accepted at the same Clinic, Uncle Mihaly greeted him saying that he knew not only his father but also his grandfather.

I worked hard and industriously at the Stomatological Clinic, even though I did not enjoy Dentistry. There were rewards, though, even in such a cold and strange place. I recall Professor Balogh standing up after I had fixed a female patient's mobile lower teeth. When I left after the demonstration he addressed the lecture room thus: "This lady has Frankl to thank. This young doctor has demonstrated a case with a long history which older doctors with greater experience could hardly accomplish". A rewarding verbal tribute.

Before closing this particular phase of my life, there is one more dear friend I must mention, namely Karcsi Csurgo. He and I had two things in common. Firstly, neither wanted to be a dentist, and secondly, we both loved and adored Anuci (as did all my colleagues, including Simon). I remember leaning out of the window of my flat at 51 Jozsef Boulevard and bemoaning with Karcsi our fate of becoming dentists. K. Csurgo had a small surgery in the centre of Budapest but his time there was short-lived, he was to die all too soon from liver cancer.

He died (in the Surgical Clinic of Professor Bakay) in an enormous, dreary floor-tiled ward, alone and deserted, a greenish-black colour but smiling to the bitter end. How much he meant to me, we were so close to each other. Karcsi Csurgo used to greet Anuci with his peculiar, deep, sonorous voice: "I kiss your hands, my dear Anuci!"

In 1932 I joined the Dental Department of the Polyclinic in Budapest under Dr Bela Simon.

Simon had organised his Department magnificently and collected his co-workers brilliantly. He found talented people from all branches of dentistry because Jewish doctors were accepted nowhere else. He had a sharp intellect and a clear head, but he never forgot his own interest. I, as a romantic character, fell in love with him immediately and respected him intensely. The Department was unified in one matter only: the

41

adoration of Bela Simon. He gave advice to everyone according to his or her practical and scientific work. Besides treating patients, he attached great emphasis to scientific studies, publications in Hungarian, and mainly in foreign papers.

The spirit - as in many other communities - was far from uniform. There were two camps: one of K.'s, the other of B. I belonged to B., who was Assistant Professor in the Stomatological Clinic before he came over to the Department. Once he came over to me to supervise my work whilst I was busy with the root treatment of an upper second incisor. The nerve was already removed from the root canal and when B. looked into the mirror he said softly: "My dear Zolti, here, in the top corner of the cavity, some pulp tissue has been left, it should have been removed before". I never forgot his teaching. One or two years later, B. again came to me and asked softly: "Dear Zolti, I have some surgical problems, could you help me?

B. was highly respected abroad as well and, although he was Jewish, he was invited in 1933 to Hitler's Germany to deliver a lecture. In January 1945 his life's reward was to be shot in the nape of the neck by a gang of laughing Hungarian Nazis by the banks of the Danube who watched as his body floated quietly downstream in the wintry, icy water of the river. I still remember how bewitched he had been some years earlier looking at one of our lady doctors dressing herself and standing in her blue slip in the Department's small dressing room.

The leader of the other group was K., who had already worked in the Department in Rothman's time. K. was a clever, talented, rather aggressive man and, because there were a great many similarities in our temperaments, we became antagonists from the first minute. Notwithstanding that, I learnt from him the so-called 'diathermy', i.e. electrosterilisation of the root canals which I am still using now, fifty years later.

42

The Department was rather small, a dressing room, the Professor's room, a small theatre, a conservative section with ten units and a small X-ray room. Once when the theatre was occupied, I treated one of our patients who was suffering from severe inflammation of the bone marrow, two units away from where K. was working. There was a plentiful amount of pus and the smell was none too pleasant either. K. protested, intensely irritated. My father was by chance also present, and said to me that K. was entirely correct. I had to admit it to myself.

However, the embers were glowing under the ashes. K. was an assistant and I a junior trainee only, but I was never inclined to obey slavishly. Besides this, I was rather sensitive and, because I often heard some not too benevolent remarks or some innuendo from him, I used to arrive home rather upset. Anuci's dear, ever-smiling face awaited me in front of the open door and she tried to emphasize the insignificance of these nasty but childish affairs.

The situation became grave only, when, in 1933, Simon opened a competition with the theme: "Dr Armin Rothman's Scientific activities in foreign literature". It was common knowledge that K. would apply as he was the closest co-worker and pupil of Rothman. However, it was soon discovered that a second application had been presented, and nobody had the slightest idea who it was who had sent it in. It turned out, also rather too soon, that the work in its thoroughness and style, was scientifically much superior in comparison to K.'s perfunctory paper. The situation became a little bit alarming because, after Simon, K. was regarded as the second 'Head' of the Department and it would have been a great blunder if he did not win the competition. The competition had naturally been *secret* and the names of the authors were attached in sealed envelopes. And then, *marvel of marvels*, it was found out that the dissertation which was better and of an incomparably higher value, was written by the 'little Frankl', the youngest member of the whole Department

... Some solution had to be found, as Dr K. could not be humiliated.

Then came the festive meeting which the Archduchess Augusta, sister of the Kaiser and Emperor Franz Joseph attended. My father and Anuci were there too. The 'B. Simon's Award' was divided in two equal parts. First, Dr K. went to Her Excellency, bowed profoundly when receiving the Award, and then kissed the black glove on her hand. After this, I went up and when I received the Award, I shook her hand. My father did not like the Habsburgs and I was not willing to kiss their black gloves. I was later informed that K. was actually fuming with rage that Frankl merely shook hands with the Archduchess.

K. tried everything to detach himself from his Jewishness. He became converted to the Roman Catholic faith, he entertained priests at his table but, for all this, he could not avoid his fate. He was deported in 1944, and when he had been transported in the usual cattle wagon from one camp to another, he lost his mind and a Nazi guard shot him on the spot. This was the end of one of Hungary's most talented dental surgeons.

Professor Simon was all charm, full of humour and inexhaustible jokes which he repeated a hundred times and laughed at them the most. Most of the women in the Department were in a rather good position and on special terms with him, which in those days in Hungary, was natural. However, among others, Anuci always kept a proper distance from him and some years later he declared to one of his girlfriends that, of all the women in his Department, he looked at Anuci with the greatest respect and reverence.

One day a pretty, nicely dressed, little dressmaker's assistant sat in my dental chair and when I finished her porcelain fillings, I sat on the arm of the chair and both of us, smiling with full devotion, agreed to a rendezvous on Margaret Island. With a fleeting sideways glance, I became aware that my professor was watching us as he leant against the door of his room. He was smiling with self-satisfaction, thinking most probably what a success he had made with his hard-won, newly purchased, new units.

Simon wanted to strengthen the solidarity of the Department with the help of social gatherings amongst other things. These gatherings were held sometimes in his house and elsewhere at other times, for instance, one dinner was held in the famous 'Deep Water' room of the Café New York. I stood up after dinner and said that it was only right that the voices of the youngest in the present company should be heard as well. I gave a short but rather rousing speech about the activities of B. Simon. I mentioned, among other things, that scarcely had the patient sat down in the chair and opened his mouth, that the gold inlay was already laughing there inside. It was a success beyond description. The owner of the New York, a well-known theatre critic, was standing at the door of the room where we were eating and heard the lecture right through. Afterwards he went to Simon and asked him who was this very talented young man and whether he could be of any help to him. "He is a young dental surgeon and, if you would really like to help him, give him lunch in your café at half price", Simon replied. Henceforth, I had my lunch always in the elegant café, sitting on a red-cushioned chair, and the fine pastries were usually consumed by Anuci.

In 1935 I took part in a Congress in Bologna, Italy, where I delivered a lecture. Before the trip, I studied Italian rather intensively and read my paper in Italian before a crowded audience. It was received with tremendous applause lasting for several minutes and in turn brought a wide, laughing smile to Simon's face, as he watched from behind the audience. I bowed and was already starting to leave when I was pulled back by my coat because someone wanted to greet me. Of course I could not understand a word of what he was saying.

At the ball following the banquet, I informed Simon and his wife of my marriage to Anuci in December, which news was received with great enthusiasm and immediately they wrote her a congratulatory letter.

We visited a clinic and went to see the lecture room as well where I found a torch which, when switched on, showed a little red arrow which pointed to the area required. I had never seen the same before and, as I was playing with it, our female guide remarked calmly: "This young doctor must be Jewish". We visited a school and, as we were looking around we were a little surprised to see, without any special emotion, eight to ten year-old children playing and exercising with toy rifles. It was Mussolini's time but we were far from the reality of what that meant; we were only interested in 'Science'.

In 1934, I got a place in the Third Surgical Clinic as an Apprentice-Surgeon. It was my father's wish that all his three children should qualify as general surgeons besides their other specialities. Father had studied together with Professor L. Adam at University and he said to him: "Dear Professor, I would like it very much if you could take my son at your Clinic". "Send him to me, Aron!" was the answer and, from that time on, I worked in Adam's Clinic as well.

One day I was giving my first intravenous injection to a charming middle-aged woman who was terribly afraid. I promised her it would not hurt. I had withdrawn the needle a long time before she asked me anxiously "when are you going to give me the injection?" I have always had a main principle not to cause the patient pain. My other principle has been that of 'Nil nocere' (not to do any harm)! Similarly, it has always been rooted in me that in most cases the patient is right, only we do not always understand why. Sometimes we became nervous, at times we shouted at the patients when there was still no diagnosis. For instance, I once asked a male patient to roll up his left arm shirt sleeve because I had to give him the prescribed injection. He did nothing, in fact he turned his head away. I asked him again, this time with a firmer tone of voice ... still nothing happened. And it turned out that his left arm was missing! I stroked the patient affectionately, feeling terribly ashamed of myself.

My first surgery in Budapest was at 51 Rakoczi Street. I had a large ball-shaped lamp, and the arm of the drilling machine hung down like the whip-handle of a draw-well in the Hungarian 'puszta' (lowland). On the street-side wall of the house I had my plate 'Dr Frankl Zoltán, Dental Surgeon', and my first patient, who happened to stray in, was a gynaecological case. She was about 20 years old and told me she was getting married in two weeks' time and that, if her husband-to-be found out that she was no longer a virgin, he would leave her immediately. Not having a gynaecological table I made her sit in my dental chair. She put her legs apart and I saw straight away, without any laboratory examination, that she had serious gonorrhoea. I warned her to go and see a urologist without delay, for her would-be husband would not be pleased with such a wedding present! Then I explained to her that, in their moment of ecstasy, men are not entirely accountable so she should make the procedure in question rather difficult; she should compress her thighs and give a loud scream! She returned after four weeks, radiant with happiness, telling me that everything had been alright except that her husband had had a minor shock after she had given such a loud yell! My fee was that for a tooth filling!

I don't know and didn't know anything about politics; however, being Jewish, the anti-Jewish Laws which started in 1937, concerned me as much as anyone else. Notwithstanding, I lived a rather isolated existence between 1930 and 1940, as if a veil were in front of my eyes. My work, my profession, meant everything to me; from early morning till late at night and somewhat to the exclusion of my family. I was totally absorbed with the Clinics and sheltered in them. In the afternoons I continued my private practice in my surgery; I had to work for our living since, in the Clinics, I did not get any salary. Often I worked till eleven at night. To use the English expression: "I kept my head down". Things could sometimes be dangerous. For example, in Kiskunhalas, a dental surgeon with a rather good reputation had extracted a tooth for somebody and the patient died some days after the extraction. The cause of death was leukaemia, or some other disease of the blood-forming tissues (blood-dyscrasia) and had no connection with the extraction of the tooth. However, my dear father was very happy that it was not he or I who had extracted the tooth because, being Jewish, we could easily have been blamed for it.

I received my Surgery Diploma in 1936.

Professor Adam started his lectures with 'Surgery of the Head' and then went downwards from the neck to the lower extremities. When he came to the mouth he then would say: "In my Clinic, Frankl deals with the surgery of 'mouth and jaws'" ... I was twenty-eight years old! Adam also emphasized decades before the teaching of the importance of the proper occlusion of the teeth, how important a really precise performance in this territory was, that surely, all of us knew, that when a 'filling' is only a half or one millimetre higher than it should be, then how much our life and concentration is disturbed.

In the 'Outpatients' Department there was an assistant, a smiling, stocky surgeon of peasant origins who passionately liked extracting teeth. The teeth he liked to extract were usually fractured and then he would say to the patient with great conviction: "I have removed the greater part of your tooth, and Frankl will now clean out the small bits which have been left in".

Adam operated wonderfully with his small, firm, steady hands and was able to save even those patients who had been sent from other hospitals with the diagnosis 'inoperable ... cancer of the bowels'. He made all his surgical interventions under local anaesthesia and, because Simon professed the same principle, it went without saying that, from my masters I fully adopted these methods.

My first operation was a 'right hernia of the groin'; Dr S., a surgeon, assisted me. Before the operation I thoroughly studied, in the dressing room, the anatomy of the region and, when the surgery was finished, S. turned to me and asked: "Where had I been operating until now?" My father's advice: *"Take great care of anatomy"* rang even then in my ears.

In 1936, with a scholarship from the Hungarian Dental Association, I went on a study tour to Vienna and Prague. In Vienna, I visited Pichler's Kieferstation. Everyday at noon and after the operations, I always had my lunch at a nearby corner restaurant; Wiener Schnitzel with potato salad costing 1 schilling and 20 groschen.

In Prague, I learned Kostecka's method for the correction of an anomaly where the lower jaw stands in front of the upper which disturbs mastication and presents an unsightly cosmetic effect. Kostecka's method is simple and brilliant. Returning to Budapest I demonstrated this method to the Dental Association, on a corpse in the Pathological Institute and pointed out how injury to the nerves and vessels can be avoided. Later I performed this operation repeatedly and successfully in my Department.

When in 1935 I went to the Congress in Bologna, Anuci parted from me in the South Railway Station in Budapest but, in 1936 Anuci accompanied me to the World Congress in Vienna. We had been in Vienna before, on our honeymoon in 1935. We were young and cheerful. It was December and Anuci did not have any warm clothes, so we went to Kärtner Strasse, one of Vienna's most expensive streets, and found a shop with beautiful, knitted dresses in the window. Anuci tried some of them on and, in the end, found a really superb brown knitted dress. The price of it was 120 schillings, which was too expensive for us. However, I asked the people in the shop to reserve it until the following day when we would return for it. Anuci thought that I had gone mad and explained that we would not have any more money tomorrow either. I replied that there was no problem, we would go to the Casino in Baden that night and win the cost of the dress. They looked at us a little oddly in the shop but even more curiously and incredulously the next day when we turned up and paid the price easily. The Casino paid for everything. Yet, the most interesting thing was that, when we had started to leave the Casino, an employee in red and white livery approached us and, on a tray, handed over to Anuci a lot of money. We looked at him in amazement when he told us that "the Lady left a gaming-chip on the first four numbers and they have come up again". Fortune favours the brave. Anuci never again had such an elegant dress.

In 1936, our friend Frici Elbogen took us back to Austria in his father's Alfa Romeo. Near Wiener Neustadt we were nearly killed on the highway when the driver of a truck coming from the opposite direction fell asleep. If Frici hadn't reacted with lightning speed and driven off the road into a field, we would surely have been crushed to death.

At Radstadt we separated from Frici and continued our way to Grünersee up an extremely winding mountain road. The driver drove without looking at the road nor the steering-wheel, but we still arrived. We had a rendezvous with L. Tisza, who later became a famous atomic physicist, and his attractive wife. I taught Tisza javelin throwing, using a cut broken piece of wood which I thought wouldn't be much use during his research work but at the time he enjoyed it very much. His lively wife later went slightly mad.

In 1937, Professor Simon and I went walking along the Boulevard towards the Oktogon when we heard a newsboy shouting "Hetföi Hirlap!" The 'First Jewish Law' had come out. I quickly bought the paper. At that moment it did not seem to affect me. Nationalistic, full of scientific ambitions, relatively well off, like other middle-class people in Budapest, I lived for the present only. The fact that the 'First Jewish Law' would be followed by a 'Second' and a Third, did not enter my mind.

In the meantime, we lived quite happily in Budapest. I walked in the Boulevard arm in arm with B. Laszlo, Anuci and B.'s wife walked behind us. As we passed by each female we turned round to our wives and said "What a fantastic woman!" Anuci remarked only: "How modest you are!" We went to the cinema and saw Greta Garbo, Dolores del Rio, Cary Grant, Clarke Gable, Chaplin, and so on. We went to theatres as well: Sandor Guoth, Frida Gombaszogi, Jeno Torzs, Iren Varsanyi, Gizi Bajor, Artur Somlay, and Latabar. We enjoyed the cabaret with Endre Nagy, Hacsek and Sajo, and Bela Salamon, etc. We listened enraptured to Marie Anderson's *Ave Maria* in the Great Concert Hall and, as if blind, ignored completely the political storms gathering around us.

Sometimes when we finished work, at around midday we boarded a tram as far as the Elizabeth Bridge and ran to the Danube Swimming Pool, as it was known, next to the river's edge where a wooden 'open' pool had been built, with dressing cubicles and places for sunbathing provided. In the middle of this simple structure was the actual pool some 10 metres wide by 30 metres long and through which the waters of the Danube flowed. It was one of those places which will be missed forever as, with the war, it disappeared as well.

After swimming and on the way home, I used to stop, many times, in front of the entrance to the 'Hungaria', one of the big hotels situated alongside the river bank of the Danube. There, in dead silence, I would listen to the wonderful sounds coming from the violin of Imre Magyari, the leader of a gypsy band. The unforgettable melodies as they cried, melted out from Magyari's violin: "Mandulafa, Mandulafa, De keves a virag rajta ..." ("Almond tree, almond tree, How few are the flowers on it") remained everlastingly in my soul. Huberman also went to listen to him. I had no money to go into the café itself, but outside the entrance the sounds were still beautiful and, as a matter of fact, I wasn't standing alone! One mustn't forget Huberman either. We heard him in the "Varosi

Szinház" (State Theatre) sitting with Anuci, far from the stage on one of the highest steps in the balcony. Anuci sat clasping her knees with her hands, her eyes shining. She was wearing a brightly coloured tailored dress. There stood Huberman in front of the orchestra, legs apart, contorted face, playing Beethoven's Violin Concerto with such a magical art that, from ecstatic joy and pain, the tears were flowing down our cheeks and we were crying unashamedly.

We loved our everyday life and did not go anywhere where we were not made to feel welcome. We had a circle of friends with whom we talked, discussed, danced, played music and so forth, and sometimes twenty to twenty-five of us would meet in our flat. We had been, unfortunately, apolitical and, had we left the country we loved so much when we had had the time so to do, then my parents could have lived much longer. In 'Dinner Dress' we went to dances in the 'Vigado' and took part in the departmental dinners so magnificently organised by Professor Simon. He took me once in his car to the Hungarian country town of Hodmezovasarhely where he delivered a lecture on focal infection. I learnt many things from him, even seemingly unimportant things; for instance that one should not keep broken mirrors in one's surgery, etc. When our Department was authorised to teach Dentistry, it was then that I lectured on Dental and Oral Surgical Anatomy.

Meantime, we made many trips to Visegrad to the so-called BOTE-House, a tourist hostel for medical doctors, and to Janoshegy, Szentendre, Kisinocz and Esztergom, where I recall Simon bravely diving into the swimming pool. More memorable than that, though, was the time when Zoltán Kodaly, aged 72, dived into the swimming pool of Lukacs.

We never forgot the evening in a small theatre when, after the compére, Bekeffy, had made an announcement and introduced the next act, the curtain would not rise fully - it was during Hitler's time - Bekeffy poked his head out from behind the curtain and said: "Nevertheless, he will be drawn up ..." The police stood speechless but the thunderous applause didn't die away for a long, long time. He wasn't hanged; but only because he committed suicide ... For us, though, too late.

One day Simon phoned me at the surgery asking me if I would take into my care the son of the Prime Minister Kallay. His lower jaw had been broken during an extraction. J.B., a charming man and a friend of mine had tried to remove the right lower first molar. The anterior root came out but when he tried to remove the posterior root in the usual way with an elevator, the jaw broke. Considering the distinguished social position of the patient, he asked the help of his professor. Simon said that he couldn't assume the treatment as, the following day he was travelling to Lake Balaton and thus recommended that the patient be referred to me. Accordingly, the young Karolyi turned up in my surgery accompanied by his aristocratic mother. I gave him injections, removed the fractured root and, in some hours, replaced and fixed the fractured fragments, using the well-known so-called Hauptmeyer splints. The patient's mother, meanwhile, was strolling quietly up and down the waiting-room being consoled by Anuci, my wife. After the operation, we had to go and see Professor Adam, the family doctor, at the Fasor Sanatorium. Adam examined the boy and then sent him for an X-ray. The X-ray report was as follows: 'In the lower jaw no trace of fracture is visible'. Adam said only: "It is alright, old chap". Then the Prime Minister turned to me, bowed and said "Would you allow me, Professor, to take you home in my car?" I accepted the invitation.

Some years later, when I was called up for Forced Labour in Bustyahaza (Northern Hungary), Anuci wrote twice to Mrs Kallay asking for her help to set me free - it would only take one word from her to the powers-that-be. She didn't reply in either instance. For myself, whilst working with pick and shovel building an airfield at Bustyahaza, I watched the Prime Minister's 'special' train rolling past as he went hunting for deer and wild boar in the Carpathians, and when I did, I plunged my pickaxe more vigorously than usual into the hard soil!

The famous German Oral Surgeon, Professor Wassmund was visiting Budapest in 1941 and had delivered a lecture to the Hungarian Dental Association about the treatment of war injuries. That same evening I sent all my scientific publications which had been published in German, to him at the Gellert Hotel. I adored him. He invited me to dinner next evening at the Gellert. He wore the uniform of a Wehrmachtgeneral and, naturally, had no doubt of the fact that I was Jewish. This fact, however, could not break our relationship or the ardent love of our profession. We discussed nearly the whole sphere of Oral Surgery.

In 1939 in Budapest, I was called up for military service and worked as a commissioned officer in the Surgical Department of one of the military hospitals. I operated on many Polish patients as well. These soldiers took refuge in Hungary when Hitler's army overran their country. Two cases had some special interest.

The first was a short, stocky major who was in great pain. He had on his neck an enormous carbuncle which occupied his whole nape. (I have only seen similar ones during my Deportation, and they were on my overworked, starved, famished mates.) Under local anaesthetic, I opened up the whole area with two long incisions, and lifted up four heavily infiltrated lobes; I secured the removal of the purulent discharges and covered the whole infected area with gauze. When the effect of the injection ceased his pain also ceased, and he recovered completely.

The other case was an 18-year old boy. I was asleep in our flat at 4 Liszt Ferenc Square, Budapest, when, one morning at 4.30, the Duty Doctor rang me from the military hospital asking whether I would be prepared to operate on a patient with acute appendicitis. Of course I agreed instantly and by taxi I arrived at the hospital within a few minutes. The patient was lying semi-conscious, pale, and with a pulse rate of 120. When I examined him, it appeared that the case was not a simple appendicitis. The abdomen was stone-hard and very painful, even to the slightest touch. There was no doubting it, he had a serious general peritonitis and I had to intervene immediately.

Two nurses (nuns) helped me in the theatre, one assisted, the other dealt with the instruments. I opened the abdominal cavity under local anaesthesia, as usual, and made to lift out the appendix. I inserted my fingers, searched, and tried to find the appendix. However, due to the inflammation, the intestines were so closely stuck together that they presented one solid inseparable mass. I tried to separate the bowels but to no avail. I worked for more than an hour, my face dripping with sweat. I knew that the patient would die if the appendix was not removed but I also knew that there would be a military-backed disciplinary action against me if the surgical intervention was not successful. Almost at desperation point, I suddenly remembered one of Professor Adam's sayings that, when you are unable to find the appendix in its usual place, then put in two fingers from your left hand, catch the tissues which first come into your hand, grasp it with a Lumnitzer (a tweezer-like metal instrument) in your right hand and pull it out. And that will be the appendix! I closed my eyes, followed the remembered instructions and, when I opened up my eyes, there it was, lying on the sheet in front of me, a perforated, purulent-gangrenous appendix. I removed it and the nurse drained the wound with some gauze placed in a glass jar. The patient, during all this time, did not feel a thing.

I arrived back home totally exhausted and only said to Anuci that a Polish mother would now not have to wait in vain any longer for her young son. But the story didn't end there. Next morning I was informed that I had to attend, without delay, the office of the Regimental Surgeon, as the Commanding Officer of the Hospital was in attendance. He was friendly but told me that, as a civilian, I could not have known that only a professional military doctor should have been allowed to perform that operation for, if a First Lieutenant enters the hospital, then he insists that he should be operated on by a Major or a Regimental Surgeon, even if a highly qualified civilian consultant or professor doing their military service is present and able to perform a professional job of a much higher value. Otherwise, he advised me, the patient in question was well ... So came to an end one of the most difficult, and perhaps the most exciting, operations of my life.

After all this, and as a consequence of the continuously worsening anti-Jewish laws I was transferred as a common infantry-man to a military barracks. There, on my very first day, the Duty Sergeant kicked over my straw mattress (which I had rolled up so very carefully) shouting: "What is this rotten heap?" And some days' later, a Major who visited the barracks for supervision, whilst our platoon was standing in line to attention, started the investigations with the following sentence: "Those rotten Jews should step forward from the ranks!"

We were demobilised shortly after because we were found to be 'not suitable', even as ordinary soldiers. This continuous humiliation against which we could not defend ourselves cracked our resistance and self-esteem. Poland had fallen, the war had started against the Soviet Union and with it the Forced Labour period began.

CHAPTER FIVE

Working Among The Tyrants

On June 25th 1942 I was ordered to go immediately to Domony. We prepared a rucksack and Anuci accompanied me to the little village in the vicinity of Budapest. As we went down the stairs from our flat in Ferenc Liszt Square, I gashed the back of my left hand on a jagged piece of metal on the handrail. We bandaged it with a handkerchief but it took some time to heal, in fact I still have a thin white scar to show, even after 50 years. In Domony there was total confusion and nobody knew where they were or what they were supposed to do. In one small room a malicious man who called himself 'Doctor' performed the medical re-examination. I had taken with me some X-rays made from my earlier lung-infection and went in to see the 'doctor' to ask for my exemption. In just a few minutes I was kicked out. One of my best friends, B. Laszlo was there and we teamed up. Next day we were ordered into cattle wagons which then headed off towards the north of the country. From time to time my mates climbed up to look through a small gap to see which way the train was headed. Was it straight to the north via Kassa to the Ukraine (which everyone dreaded, as it meant certain death), or again, was it diverted to somewhere unknown? Fortunately, it turned North East and we came to a halt in Bustyahaza.

On the way it was forbidden to write home but, on the initiative of L. Urbach, the famous inventor of the Matra Motorcycle, we set about writing letters anyway. These letters soon got into the hands of the crew who escorted us. These soldiers were primitive, illiterate and merciless, and our letters were handed immediately to the Lieutenant Commandant of the company. For breaking the rules, Urbach's hands were tied together and he was hung for two hours, from a branch so that only his toes touched the ground. Laszlo and I had to sit on the ground, our hands and feet tightly bound. Actually, as we were motionless anyway, it was not so awkward and, in any event, they set us free early. Our quarters were in a large wooden building, a timber warehouse the size of half a football ground. The floor was wooden plank, under which there was a hole some five or six metres deep. During the nights it was very chilly, the cold coming partly from beneath, and partly from the harsh North East wind outside howling through the wooden walls. B. Laszlo had a warm sleeping bag lined with cotton or wadding. Mine was lined only with some artificial material ... Anuci had been cheated in the Terez Boulevard in the same way as soldiers going to the front in the First World War, by unscrupulous tradesmen, Jews amongst them, who sold the soldiers unlined laced boots, some with paper soles! We felt thoroughly miserable and, in the evenings before lying down, we put on all the clothes we had, pullovers, winter coats, etc.

In the mornings we fell into line and went to build an 'airfield', a fenced off area of more than ten square kilometres. We carried spades, hacks, shovels and pickaxes, and began to level off the rough, stony scrub area and, when we had levelled one section, were moved on to start another, working from morning till night. The whole thing, of course, was a transparent deception: Jewish men of military age had to be removed from Budapest or from their homes. There were two companies in Bustyahaza, Nos. 101/39 and 101/40 and these were the last two companies which were *not* sent to the Ukraine. The possibility that we might be sent, though, filled us with fear. Slowly the situation became clearer. Commandant Szollar ordered a line-up in front of our barracks to select the doctors amongst us. B. Laszlo, standing so upright in his knickerbockers and jacket, was selected and so was I as surgeon and dental surgeon.

In the middle of the camp there were some small huts, one of which we marked out as a Surgery. We built a little fireplace. We had plenty of wood and were able then to sterilise the instruments in a mess tin. We had bandages and medicines as well. An older, shortish mate of ours, Fani, became our assistant. I made a small wooden box for myself and we painted a red cross on both sides of it. In it I carried my instruments, cotton wool, etc.

The Company Commandants had separate quarters and I was called one afternoon to Szollar's quarters because he had terrible toothache. I rushed over, examined him, and diagnosed an acute inflammation of one of the lower molars; the tooth had to be removed. I went back to our 'surgery', sterilised a syringe, a needle and forceps and returned then to Szollar. I injected him and extracted the tooth. He didn't feel a thing and thanked me for it. The intervention was simple; however, its success meant a great deal to us - after all, he could have had us shot. In fact, his manner became substantially friendlier.

The officers were bored. One morning, Szollar asked for me and started to chat about the arts, paintings, Italy and so on. Alongside the surgery there were other 'offices': Administration, Workshop for the mechanics and, most important of all, the Cook House. Occasionally we got excellent beef stew for dinner and sometimes, in the mornings before we started work, Mr Larcsuk, the Camp guard, would give us titbits like scrambled egg. Briefly, we were not starving, and for this we had our Commanders to thank, as they also preferred to eat well.

In our billet, Dr Laszlo slept between myself and Dr Galocsi. One night Laszlo woke me up saying that Galocsi had had a heart attack and that he, Laszlo, had prepared a lifesaving injection and he wanted me to tie down Dr Galocsi's upper arm so that he could see the vein by the light of his torch. Bela Laszlo was the finest man I had ever known and it was the first time that he yelled at me loudly and impatiently because I was still half asleep and did not hold down the vein properly and quickly enough. The injection worked and Galocsi regained consciousness, but it was imperative that he was rushed to hospital. However, only the Ruthenian doctor who lived in the village nearby was authorised to ask for an ambulance and so I immediately went to our Commandant for permission to call on the doctor. Permission received, I jumped on a bike and, in near darkness cycled down an unmade track to the village, some few kilometres away. The doctor turned out to be a rather repulsive man but, when I explained that I had come with my Commandant's permission, he asked for an ambulance. The ambulance men soon arrived and, when Galocsi was aboard, the question arose as to who should accompany him to the hospital in Munkacs. It meant quite a lot to us to leave the camp, if only for a short time. Bela and I looked at each other and then I suggested that fate should be decided by 'heads or tails'. Bela won and he accompanied Galocsi ... there was a little humour left in us, even during these difficult times. Galocsi recovered, due to the prompt action taken by Laszlo and, after the liberation, he became the Director of the Peterfi Sandor Hospital. It is the irony of fate that, in 1957, after the Revolution was put down, he signed one of the necessary authorisations allowing me to depart for Italy to deliver a lecture, in reality, to leave the country.

In the camp we settled into a routine and, with some bribery, the tension between us and our guards became less. But, it was still captivity. In the meantime, the so-called 'Tree Trunk Club' was established. There was a place in the compound where some tree trunks had been carelessly stockpiled and it was here that the intellectuals of our group gathered in the evenings for discussions, gossip and lectures. It was an important spiritual event, in contrast with the day's long, physical work. All the vicissitudes and hardship could not yet kill our spirit. While Peter, the art historian, and Gottsegen, the heart specialist, stood guard at the railings, we argued with each other about the most complicated questions of Art and Philosophy.

Letters from home were, naturally, the greatest joy for us. I was always inclined to depression, mainly about financial matters, and, in the prison camp, only Anuci's boundless optimism kept my spirits up. I soon learnt all her letters off by heart and brought most of them home! "We have to pay for our wonderful life up to now, and for what may come". "I love you and I live only so to love you".

Then came the reports about my lovely little son, Andris who, though only four years old, stood manfully by his mother, sharing her sorrows and delights.

It caused the greatest of rejoicing when our wives were allowed to visit us. It was a long, hard journey from Budapest but they all came. They stayed a very short while. We sat on the ground, holding each other's hands and eating some of the food brought from home. We spoke about everything and nothing. Andris and my dear parents were the main subjects. From one part of the camp one could see the trains and, in the late afternoon when Anuci's train rolled home, she stood in her greenish-brown jersey, on the steps of a carriage, with her combed hair streaming in the wind, holding her rucksack on her left shoulder, and waving to me with her right hand. Later she told me that she had seen me waving as well.

B. Gyorgy discovered a public bath in the village of Bustyahaza, a so-called Jewish religious bath, 'mikve'. We went there once a week if we were lucky. After the bath we drank marvellous coffee and ate fantastic cakes made by the kind woman who was in charge of the bath. It cost hardly anything. She informed us that the Jews from the neighbouring villages had already been deported.

One day it struck me that there were too many cases of diarrhoea in the camp. It turned out that, after close inspection, a sloping path from the latrines led to one of the wells which supplied us with drinking water. I had permission to telephone Anuci immediately, to send us a reagent to trace the nitrite which could prove whether the contamination came from the latrine or not. Szollar, himself a hypochondriac, urged me to perform the investigation as soon as possible. Anuci was very happy that we could talk for a little bit. We used every opportunity to outwit the rules, and I asked Anuci to tell my brother Jozsi to send the reagent, which he did by return of post. Szollar was really rather moved when the colour of the water turned red due to the effect of the reagent, i.e. the result was positive. The well was shut down, the diarrhoea disappeared, and our prestige grew accordingly.

Another important event in our lives was when we used to bathe in a nearby brook called the *Talabor*. We marched down in military formation and dipped and washed ourselves happily in the ice-cold water. The Talabor was an extremely rapid mountain stream, no deeper than 50 cms but so strong and swift that we could hardly stand up in it. During our swim there were always cries of "Catch it! Hold it!". So that the people further down could catch the soap which the swift running water had snatched from our hands. We were fresh and clean, and free from lice. Then came autumn and winter. It became too cold to use the Talabor.

Meantime, rumours persisted that we might be sent to the Ukraine after all, but they always died away and we continued our work in our small hut. The cooks even made love through the fence with the local gypsy girls who could be persuaded to do anything for a few scraps of food.

Then Szollar was relieved, and his replacement was a kinder, older commandant. I once had to treat his wife in Bustyahaza; she was bored and wanted mainly to chat with me. We started a long conversation during which I told her that her eyes were like the colour of the sea in a painting by Velasquez! Unfortunately, I had selected the wrong artist for, on the next occasion she declared that Velasquez had never painted the sea. I tried to convince her that, never mind the painter, the colour of the French and Spanish Mediterranean

Sea is a wonderful blue! Following our demobilisation, she became a faithful patient of mine in Budapest.

Mid-December we moved from the timber yard to a small village near Huszt where we were put up in wooden huts. Gottsegen sat calmly on a small bench while I removed one of his upper molar teeth.

One afternoon we visited a Jewish family in a nearby village who were still left undisturbed in their home. We chatted in their warm room, five of us and as many girls. They saw us out and strolled with us a little way in the darkening starry night. We embraced and kissed them goodbye, our repressed passions bursting out. God only knows what happened to them later.

At last the day of our demobilisation arrived. We travelled back to Domony where we spent another night. The next day in Budapest I was able to embrace Andris, who jumped at me from the door, almost knocking me off my feet. I was able too, to hug Anuci... It was the 7th January 1943.

Some weeks later, a new summons arrived for labour service in the then so-called anti-aircraft defence: first, to a fire station in Tass Vezer Street, and then to a Sanatorium in Budakeszi. Finally, and until the end of the autumn in 1944, to the headquarters of the Ambulance stations in Marko Street.

Meanwhile in Kiskunhalas my dear Mother and Father were taken to the ghetto. For a short time Father could still go to work; then this was prohibited. The rest followed very quickly: soon they were taken by lorry to the railway station where they were crammed into cattle wagons. On the way they saw the family house for the last time.

At the end of June 1944 we received a postcard from Szeged from an acquaintance informing us that my parents had been deported to Austria on the 28th June. Father had suggested they commit suicide, he had sufficient morphine on him, but Mother replied: "I have been working all my life to bring up my children, now I would like to enjoy them a little". First they were taken to Wiener-Neustadt, then to a manufacturing plant in Rosenau.

All these events, of course, we heard later. For a long time we heard nothing about them. Then, one day, sometime in July, I received a postcard with an Austrian postage stamp. It was from my parents. I read it with trembling hands and tearful eyes. They asked for warm clothes. I could not put up with the thought of Mother being cold and shivering, so I rang Anuci. I told her I was going up to Buda, to the Gestapo, to ask for permission to send a parcel. Anuci begged me not to, for we all knew that no Jew or 'leftist' person who went up there ever came back. "I will go", I answered and put down the receiver.

I took a taxi and asked the driver to take me up to the Gestapo. He looked at me for a long time, but I got into his car and he started off. The Commandant, Obersturmführer Danneker, was sitting behind his desk. I jumped to attention, told him who I was and that I had come to ask for permission to send a parcel of clothes to my parents working at an Austrian factory. He pointed to another table, told me to take a yellow-coloured form and fill it in. He then signed and stamped it. I started for the door when he called after me. My heart missed a beat. Then, half smiling, he handed the signed admission card to me saying: "You will need this to get out of the building". I thanked him and left. The taxi driver looked at me again with some surprise and then we started homeward. Later, the whole thing seemed to have been so simple. Years later, I heard in London that Danneker was a war criminal.

When Anuci saw me, words failed her. She could not believe her eyes when she saw and read the Gestapo's written permission. Quickly she made up a parcel of the finest clothes and underwear; she even put a Kohinoor B pencil into one of Father's pockets - he liked writing with them so much.

I was still in Marko Street when the situation became suddenly very grave. Margit (Mámá) our domestic help, took Andris down to her brother in Jaszbereny where we hoped he would be safer. Not long after this, though, we received a telephone message saying, however, that Andris should be brought back instantly because, according to a new decree, in a few days time all Jewish children were to be rounded up and collected. Wearing my overall, with my armband marked 'Légó-orvos' ('Ambulance-doctor') I dashed to the Headquarters of the Gendarmerie in Budapest and begged the Colonel in charge that he should take steps to see to it that my son should not be deported from Jaszbereny. He told me that I shouldn't imagine they were 'child-killers' but I continued with my plea until finally he phoned the officer in charge at the Gendarmerie in Jaszbereny instructing that "the little Frankl should be left alone". That evening Margit brought Andris home. Anuci and I waited for them at the Western Railway Station.

All the other children were deported.

On October 15th, 1944 we heard Governor Horthy's radio proclamation about Hungary's separate peace treaty and her exit from the war. Anuci phoned me. The Germans were supposed to be packing and getting ready to leave. We were pleased, of course, but after so many disappointments we could not relax completely. Somehow it didn't smell right ... A few hours later we were lined up in the courtyard of the Ambulance Station in Marko Street just as an officer arrived in Arrow Cross or SS uniform. Our own Christian Commander appeared and said something to him. The other officer drew his revolver and shot him in the leg without saying a word. That was the beginning ...

Szálasi and his Arrow Cross men had taken charge, and news began to stream in about their cruelties. We were so filled with fear that even through the window we dreaded to see the 15- and 16-year old lads approach our building, in single file, carrying rifles and wearing Árpád bands (Hungarian Arrow Cross armbands).

I had to find a haven for my wife Anuci and my son Andris. I took them by ambulance to Professor Adam's Surgical Clinic where I had worked for many years. A few days later I got a call telling me that Anuci had to leave the Clinic because of the raids. At first, Anuci tried to return to our flat in Ferenc Liszt Square, but the concierge would not let her into the building. So she came to stay with me at the Ambulance Station. Dr Lederer, my colleague at the Ambulance Station, suggested that I should have her transferred to the Alice Weiss Hospital, and Dr Pista Csillag arranged this. The Alice Weiss Hospital gave refuge to many of the doctors' wives and children under false pretences.

Again, a few days later, I got another call from the Adam Clinic to say that my son Andris was well, after his operation. What operation? I was startled. It turned out that Professor Adam had called them from his hiding place in Buda telling them to take little Frankl's appendix out because the Arrow Cross men were going to take everyone away who was not a post-operative patient. Poor Andris, he screamed and resisted. After all there was nothing wrong with him.

A few days later I received another phone call to say that I must get Andris out of the Clinic because even the post-op children were being taken away. One of my colleagues hid him with his own son overnight and the next morning I had him taken to Anuci in the Alice Weiss Hospital. The Director of the Hospital told me that he would keep Andris there if I obtained a 'Swiss Pass' for his son. So I went to the so-called Glass House and got a pass for him. I was able to evade the bloodthirsty Arpad patrols because of my military cap and my ambulance overall with a red cross on it.

As always, Anuci remained cool-headed and soon they assigned her to operate their switchboard. These were difficult times, and they were getting harder. Rumours came flooding in, one after another and, in the end, they all turned out to be true. But we remained naïve and, while they were deporting the Jews from Ujpest, we were saying that it was inconceivable that it could ever happen in Budapest.

Air raids, sorties, and whenever possible a brief stop at the Hospital were the order of the day.

One afternoon, I was lying on the upper bunk when one of our dear friends, Elek Barna, a famous painter, came in to see me. "I'm going to find my wife Anci. They dragged her off from the brickworks this morning and got her marching towards Austria". That's all he said. Anci was slim and fragile and was probably lost, with hundreds of others suffering from diarrhoea, before reaching the border.

––––––––––––

We suddenly received our orders to pack for departure after lunch on November 27th. Like the others, I tried to stuff everything possible into my rucksack: a spoon, a mess bowl, two cups, shirts, underpants, socks, etc. I was wearing the ski boots given to me in the thirties by an old friend, Dr Frici Elbogen. It was most important for me to pack all the *oral surgical instruments* to hand in my separate little medical bag: a mirror, tooth forceps, curettes, pincers, surgical forceps, scalpel, whetstone, winter-type elevators, gauze, cotton, sulphonamides, analgesics, etc. I had originally taken these along to the Ambulance Station, consciously, or perhaps by instinct. I had prepared them with great care. I also took with me my sheepskin-lined leather jacket, a gift from my father. I quickly phoned Anuci to let her know that we were being taken to the military barracks on Arena Avenue. We were ordered to fall in and began our march. At the Western Railway Terminal we got so mixed up with the huge crowd that it would have been easy to escape, but this was just a passing thought, and we marched on. We were led to a big hall on the first floor, and slept, dressed as we were, on the bare slatted wooden floor. Dr Bela Laszlo was lying next to me, just as in the labour camp in Bustyahaza.

In the morning, black coffee and bread were handed out. Early in the afternoon they suddenly ordered us to line up in the courtyard. A police officer was running up and down in front of us hollering like a maniac. Dr Lederer was standing in the front row next to me; he could hardly breathe. Suddenly, I snapped out of the line and froze to attention in front of the police officer and said: "I humbly report that this doctor should be allowed to step aside from the column because he suffers from severe pulmonary disease and will die after just a few steps". The officer looked at me and signalled that Dr Lederer should step out of the line. That is how I repaid my debt to him for having Anuci taken to the Hospital. Although he died a few weeks later, I still saved him from a lot of trouble.

We got going, out through the gate and then along Arena Avenue towards the railway station in Jozsefvaros. I carried my heavy rucksack, and the heavy rucksack carried me forward. There were about 1,800 of us and we were escorted by only five or six middle-aged and indifferent rifle-carrying privates. We could have 'done them in' easily, but who would have dared to think of that? As we marched past Anuci's Hospital I was thinking where I could go, who would take me in? I concluded sadly that, after thirteen years of residence in Pest, there was not one among the thousands of patients and friends to whom I could turn. I looked back once and saw that my orthopaedist colleague, Dr Tibor Grosz, wearing a hat and winter coat but no rucksack, had elegantly stepped out of the formation and quietly wandered off towards the Liget (Park). I found out after my return from deportation that he was subsequently executed together with his wife and child on a park bench in the Liget, by some Arrow Cross men.

The cattle trucks stood gaping and empty at the railway station and we stood in front of them. I noticed a good-looking, elegant young man in a winter coat and wearing a soft, flat hat, with a book in his hand; one after another men were rushing over to him, he was Raoul Wallenberg. In turn, I went to him to report that I only had a Swiss 'Schutzpass' but my brothers-in-law and their entire families were under Swedish protection. He leafed through his book and then told me that, unfortunately, I was not on his roster and there was nothing he could do, whereupon I started back towards the wagon. As they were helping me up into the wagon, Dr Laci Friedman shouted out that someone had dropped a satchel. I suddenly realized, with fear, that my *medical bag* was missing, and happily reached out for it. It was to turn out eventually that this simple action saved my life and the lives of many, many others. As I was trying to get into the wagon I heard Bela Laszlo shout from the front of the next wagon: "Zolti, I am here". Because he was holding up the line whilst he shouted out to me, a police officer struck him so hard in the face that he fell down. That is how we got separated. He also survived and returned home; the police officer was later hanged in Budapest. I tossed a few written lines to Anuci out of the wagon, and she received them in the Hospital within a few hours: "My Anuci, I am following my father; I shall be looking for you everywhere; take care of each other. Love Zolti". They closed and latched the door. It let out a frighteningly sad sound.

It was so crowded in the wagon that we could only stand. Occasionally someone could squat or sit for a while. Around midnight the train got going and I was suddenly overcome by such an irresistible crying fit that my comrades could barely calm me down. Meantime, the train kept going. We urinated through a gap by the door. Not until a couple of days later did they let us out at some small wayside guardhouse where they distributed bread and cheese. There were corpses covered with dark blankets lying next to the guardhouse, but we still believed that we were being transported to work in Germany. We changed trains in Sopron, and then entered Austria and arrived at Köszeg, which by then was considered, somehow, to be German territory! Rules are rules! In Köszeg they took us to a brickworks and quartered us in the basement, surrounded by a multitude of pipes. I noticed a tap and immediately undressed, and when stark naked, thoroughly washed myself in cold water. "See", said one of the others, "That's the way to prevent being lice-ridden". Twenty-four hours later I was just as lice-ridden as everyone else.

Our group of thirty-five physicians were assigned a small room, four by six metres, and we had just enough space for all of us to lie down, and my spot was next to Zsiga Barta who was somehow automatically elected to be our leader. I asked him to let me work with him as a surgeon because I had my surgical and dental instruments with me. It did not take much persuasion, particularly when someone asked who our surgeon would be. My colleague, Erno Balázs blurted out that only Frankl could do it because he was the only one to bring his tools.

Shortly after this episode I was called away to the cook's quarters where someone was ill. When I finished my business there, someone stuck a piece of meat into my hand. Upon returning to our room, I called over to Ernö who was lying in the opposite corner, and tossed half of the meat to him which he caught in mid-air.

From that time on, we marched out every day from dawn to dusk, to dig trenches against the Russian tanks - without much effect as it turned out. Black coffee, bread and soup made up our daily diet. At the beginning I was swinging the pickaxe and shovel with great elan, but the swinging of the pickaxe gradually slowed. We also dug our latrines - there was a distance of thirty to forty metres between the Men's and Women's where we squatted and held diarrhoea contests!

On the evening of December 24th, Zsiga Barta and I took a stroll to urinate into a puddle near the factory. We looked up into the crystal-clear starry sky and asked each other whether we would ever go home. The stars did not respond.

At the beginning of 1945 we were moved into paper and canvas tents pitched on a sloping field. Water was seeping into the already wet soil and often it was so cold at night that we just urinated there, in the middle of the tent.

By now there was a serious need for medical help; a small 'community' of physicians and their helpers had developed. Bit by bit they put together a wooden platform, so that it was no longer necessary to sleep on the bare ground. They even conjured up a stove-like contraption and, miracle of miracles, we even had warm water occasionally and we could sterilize our instruments in a mess-tin. There were two of us doing the medical work: Zoli Ujhelyi took care of the medical cases, and I did the dental and surgical ones; between us we gradually got rid of the lice. By the way, one could recognise lice by the characteristic popping sound made when you picked the soft thing up from the itchy spot, and squeezed it between your thumbnails! The black-clothed guards from western Hungary were so afraid of lice that they did not dare enter the tents. These men could compete in brutality with the SS. On one occasion a beautiful blonde boy of seventeen was made to dance before them in the area between the kitchen and their quarters. "Tanzen, tanzen, schneller, schneller!" ("Dance, dance, faster, faster!") they screamed, and then turned him into a sieve with a round of bullets. I walked back to the tent in silence, feeling dreadfully sad. Another time, I heard a shot while in my tent and almost immediately I was rushed to another one some thirty metres away where a man had been shot in the stomach. He was moaning and half conscious. I ran back to return with a morphine-filled syringe and gave him the injection. By now he was unconscious and his scrotum was steadily swelling with blood - some big vessels must have been struck by the bullet. Exceptionally, the Commander did come over to say that he would look into what had happened. What had happened in fact was that the poor man had gone outside his tent to hang up some clothing that he had washed and, thirty metres away, a German guard, out of sheer boredom, had decided to use him for target practice.

We were full of fear, but the greatest dread took hold of us when we saw the Hungarian military police pass our camp on horseback. They were the embodiment of the greatest horror.

I don't quite know how, but we always had enough medicine and bandages. My whetstone was with me, the same one I was to use later in my Harley Street surgery in London. I began every morning, at 5.30, honing my surgical scalpels; they had to be extremely sharp as we were forced to operate without anaesthesia. Blistered heels, purulent wounds, furuncles and carbuncles, were the most common problems. How many times was it necessary to expose surgically gigantic, necrosed, purulent areas, and clean out pus and necrotic tissues beneath the elevated lobes (which extended over the entire back) using 15-20 cm cross-cuts? Use them I did, employing the techniques I had learned at the Adam Clinic. The boys and girls never even budged. These interventions would have been life-saving had not the combined effects of starvation, physical exhaustion, depression, lack of antiseptic agents and total absence of vitamins destroyed our patients.

From January and February onwards more and more perished. They did not suffer. They went to bed in the evening and by morning they were asleep forever.

Another morning, a young girl complained about a toothache which was driving her mad. She was terribly frightened. One of her upper left premolars had an acute inflammation. I assured her that she would not feel any pain, and propped her head against the side of the tent pressing my left thumb against the nerve under the socket of the eye that supplies the tooth. As she cautiously opened her eyes, the little girl began to cry with delight, seeing the tooth in the jaws of the pincers. All this is routine procedure for the

Chinese but, to succeed, it is essential to gain the total confidence of the patient.

It was important for me to keep the spirit of my comrades high. I regularly made the rounds of the tents, to those who no longer had the strength to march out to work, lying there on damp, soggy straw. "Don't let yourselves fall apart, this can't last much longer!" I told them.

During one of my rounds, a short man of about 35 stopped in front of me, pulled up his shirt and said: "Look here, Doc, this is how skinny I am, but otherwise I feel fine! Do you think that I can make it back home? I must be able to go home, you know, because I have an exceptionally talented son, a pianist, and I want to raise him to be a world-famous artist". I looked at him, but all I saw was a skeleton; the ribs stood out through the taut skin on his tight, narrow chest, there was not even a microscopic quantity of fat around them. He just stood there, his shirt raised, waiting for some consolation. "Shut your mouth, my friend!" I said to him while patting his ribs. "How can you ask such a stupid question? You can see for yourself that you are skinny, but otherwise healthy, and you'll make it home and you'll be able to teach your son". He was calm as he took his eyes off me with a barely visible smile on his face, while letting his shirt drop. I went to see him again the following day. He was lying there quietly, dead. His neck, and the area around his right lower jaw were tremendously swollen, but there was no sign of suffering on his calm and peaceful face. His son did become a world-famous artist and, after much hesitation, I once told him, in the lobby of the Budapest Conservatory, of my encounter with his father.

When the first doctor, a young, smiling, thin paediatrician died, we accompanied him to the camp gate, dragging the cart with his corpse and those of fifteen or twenty others on it. We even said a prayer, the "El mole rahamim ..." (Merciful God) but after that we were falling so fast, one after another, that no one followed the cart anymore. There was a pathologic anatomy professor among us - I was once his student - he left too. Twenty-eight among the thirty-five doctors died.

There was a lot of diarrhoea but we did have paper for quite some time; however, it was when pages from Hebrew prayer books first began to appear in the latrine that I became desperately sad, and for the first time a sense of hopelessness took hold of me. At that time the Jewish State had not come into existence and my mother had taught us to consider the Hebrew prayer books holy and to kiss them.

I really did not have much time to think, as I worked from early in the morning until late into the evening, virtually without a break. But this was my duty and, after all, I did not have to march to dig trenches. When the others returned after a day's labour, they were exhausted to the point of numbness.

I never starved but I never had enough to eat either. When we laid down at night, close to each other on the wooden platform, I closed my eyes and recalled my mother's cooking: the breakfasts, lunches, snacks and suppers in Kiskunhalas, bread and butter, Wiener schnitzels, goulash, pureed lentils, fried chicken, stuffed cabbage, sponge cake and so on ... In this way I never went to sleep hungry and I probably smiled when after a day's worries and work, I fell asleep at last., I never woke up feeling hungry either.

After work one evening, they ordered us to line up. We were then informed that every fifth one in our group would be executed because someone had escaped. After an hour of standing in line they announced that only every tenth one would be executed. I began to count whether I or my friend standing next to me, would be tenth; but then the doctors were ordered to go to their tents and they let us all go back to sleep although that wasn't easy.

Spring began to arrive and I started chasing people out of their tents. Those who stayed inside were a lost cause; we simply referred to them as suffering from the syndrome 'Straw Disease'; they had resigned themselves to death by way of stale air of the tent, the stench of the urine, the faeces and the rotten straw.

The atmosphere somehow became tense on March 22nd and, on the 23rd, they sorted out the sick who could not march - they would be transported separately - and the rest of us were marched off as fast as we could go. We heard dull thuds along the road and suspected that the Russians were approaching. Suddenly, we heard a long round of machine-gun fire. We later learned that they had killed all the sick whom they had sent off on a different road. Someone told us that the patients who could not be moved remained in one of the tents. They loaded down the tent rims with dirt and clay and stuck a tube through them from the exhaust pipe of a car, to gas the ones inside. Other than these, twelve people stayed behind to clean up and put things in order. When they had finished, the Commander had them lined up for a headcount. He counted thirteen. One of the men had scraped the dirt out from under the tent and managed to crawl out. When the Commander demanded to know who was not present at the first line-up he stepped forward. The Commander drew his revolver and shot him without a word.

The column then began its march from Kőszeg to Mauthausen through Austria, doing thirty to forty kilometres a day, from dawn to late evening. The guards - from different villages - were changed every morning so that they could rest and feel fresh. They chased us on shouting: "Ge'mah, Ge'mah, los!" We had black coffee and a piece of bread in the morning, and some soup in the evening. We shuffled along. Ahead of us a woman suddenly squatted down to urinate right in front of us, as it was forbidden to step out of the column. Pali Koltai, Ujlaki and I led our group. We were marching downhill near Eisenerz one afternoon when all of a sudden a detachment of SS attacked us with machine guns from the side. The bullets were sprayed everywhere. I can still hear the whistle of one as it passed by me, a few centimetres from my ear. At the same moment, my dental technician friend,

K.T., was shot in the head and hit the ground; he was marching right in front of me. When he raised his head slightly, they crushed it with the butt of a rifle.

"Drei in einer Reihe, drei in einer Reihe ...!" "Three in a row"... The SS kept repeating the cry as we kept running down the hill like cattle chased by cowboys. They made us stop at the bottom of the hill as, by then, it was dark and cold and we were shivering, while perspiration was pouring off our bodies. Later, I collapsed in some little room but, before I could sleep, I heard the sound of a radio from a nearby room and managed to glean that the Allies were rapidly advancing. Next morning we were told that the attack by the SS detachment would be investigated. Who knows, perhaps, with the help of the Vatican, they were later accommodated somewhere in Latin America, as it was rumoured in Budapest. The behaviour of the Vatican was not one bit better than the brutality of the Spanish Inquisition, and there is no such God who could forgive this, despite all the prayers of the perpetrators. Then, as if nothing had happened, we marched on ...

One day, we were given large portions of stew. We carefully guarded our mess bowls and spoons, because the spoon was the key to life. As soon as I had polished off the unexpected feast, one of the men needed a huge abscess on his hand opened, with a scalpel first dipped in alcohol, and then burnt. An SS officer who had watched the procedure signalled me to follow him. He led me to the cook at the head of the mess line and ordered him to give me another portion. Much later, in Budapest, that man proudly showed his scar to me.

At other times, our luck was not so good, and we were always hungry. Whilst resting one night, I noticed in the light coming from the guardhouse, that something was being tossed onto the trash pile from large containers. Hunger is a powerful master, so I sneaked over to investigate what it could be. It turned out to be potato peelings, and still warm. They must have peeled them with a machine because, thank God, a lot of potato was left on them. I gathered up what I could and Koltai and one of the women made some soup out of them. The soup was terribly sandy, but not a drop was left over.

The nights were still very cold and we always slept on the wet grass, huddled together, men and women, to keep each other warm; everyone wore all their clothes. I was saved, thanks to my father's sheepskin-lined jacket.

Shortly before reaching the outskirts of Graz, a sweet little girl took about twenty steps to the side to relieve herself. A guard shouted then fired at her immediately; the bullet went through her thigh and her female companions helped her back into the line. The bullet had not struck bone and we took care of the wound. A rest period was ordered and I went off to find a pharmacy in town, because I knew that she could not be saved without a tetanus shot. The pharmacist, to whom I told the story, was very decent and, without much questioning, gave me the serum. I rushed back to boil a syringe in a mess-bowl and gave her the injection. She was able to hobble along with us, while using a stick and getting some support. She, too, returned to Budapest.

Gradually we got started again and, as we were passing a small house with a garden, I asked the little Austrian girl leaning on the gate whether she could give us something sweet. She stared at me wide-eyed as if she had not understood me, but she ran into the house and returned with a little bit of jam in the bottom of a glass jar. She could have had no idea how much we enjoyed this unexpected treat. The jar was only a third full, but it lasted a long time because we only took a tiny taste each.

Spring was slowly breaking through and, in spite of our misery, we could not help but notice how beautiful the country around us was. Our rucksacks were becoming heavier and heavier and more and more discarded belongings were gathering on the grassy strip along the road. I threw away nothing, but whenever we had to get started it was always very difficult to pick up my rucksack; I had got used to carrying it.

We were hungry. Some of the men were picking up snails from the rocks along the edge of the road. I was taught by my friend, Matyi Szekely, a dental technician, how to suck out the juices from the stalks of wheat. Matyi and I became close friends. He helped me get my pack on my back in the mornings and showed me the photograph of his gorgeous wife, who was from Kolozsvar. At that time, we did not know that she would not return from Auschwitz. Lying in the grass during our rest stops, we picked out the stalks of green wheat and yellow flowered rape from amongst the poppies, and then we would suck them diligently.

About a day and a half before reaching Mauthausen, our road merged with another to form a 'V', and then continued as one. Shortly after passing this junction, we heard some amazing shrieks, followed by persistent crying and sobbing. For the first time in months we were listening to cries of joy! One of the men, Mayer, who was marching along with us along the left branch of the 'V', had met his wife who was being chased along the right branch. They embraced each other and then continued their journey with their arms tightly linked. Meanwhile, more and more of the men ran out to the fields along the road to scratch out some potatoes left over from the year before. The guards shouted at them repeatedly, and finally fired a volley at them. Those who were still alive rushed back into the line. All I could see was that Mayer had collapsed directly ahead of me. I ran to his side and, as I lifted his head, I saw that he had been hit in the chin by a bullet. It had broken his lower jaw and knocked out three of his front teeth. I placed a pressure bandage over the wound and fixed the lower jaw to the skull by wrapping the bandage round and round the head. While doing this we were forced repeatedly to bend down to avoid the bullets flying over our heads. Once more, as if nothing had occurred, Mayer took his wife's arm again and continued the march. Mayer kept talking and his every step was marked by a drop of blood on the road. I screamed at him: "Shut your bloody mouth, because you're going to bleed to death before we reach Mauthausen". He did shut up, and the bleeding stopped at once. We knew nothing about Mauthausen except that they told us that we were being taken to a nice new camp. But, when I asked an almost human-looking guard about it as he passed by, his only reply was: "Entsetzlich" ("Dreadful, Terrible, Horrible").

We arrived at Mauthausen on April 14th 1945. We did not even see a gate but were herded into a bare courtyard with greyish-black soil, to spend the night there. I learned at this time that Ernö Balázs had collapsed and died about 100 metres from Mauthausen. His heart could not take any more, but at least he did not suffer further. Next morning, we saw some kind of building on one side and some trees, but there wasn't much of a chance to see anything else as they pushed us into a gigantic paper and canvas tent where we lay down on the ground. Another group arrived from Austria 24 hours later, and I went up to the top of a mound and began to shout out whether anyone had met Dr Frankl's family from Kiskunhalas. And indeed, someone did respond: one of the daughters of the quilt maker, Krausz from Halas, whose group had been working in Austria. She even brought a little reserve food with her in a small basket that she was trying very hard to protect. It was, of course, stolen from her a few days later in Gunskirchen. The girl wasn't quite herself but she told me that she had been in my father's group and that they had been transported in a Pullman car! My father had been transferred to a different place entirely and the Pullman car was, in fact, a cattle wagon, as I later discovered.

I was walking around the camp the next morning when Mayer's wife approached me and said that she had heard that I was a well-known oral surgeon from Budapest and she asked me to help her husband. Crushed by the events and surprised, I looked at her sadly and replied: "My dear lady, don't you see that we are entirely surrounded by death? Give me some time, at least until tomorrow to think about it''. She left me with tears in her eyes. I began to assemble some 'instruments' for the repair of his fractured mandible. I had been studying Professor Wassmund's book on the freehand treatment of the broken jaw caused by a bullet, whilst serving as a forced-labour air-raid emergency physician at the Sanatorium in Budakeszi in 1944 (I still have the book), so I knew what to do.

We managed to get together everything that was essential. We had dental technicians in our group who, just as I had done, had automatically taken along with them some of their tools, including pincers and nippers. Mrs Mayer scratched the ground to dig out a piece of thick aluminium wire, and I pulled out a piece of electrical wire that was dangling from the wall of our barracks. After the wire was stripped of its insulation we had our fine wire for binding each individual tooth to a thick metal band, in this case to the aluminium, which was adjusted to the upper and lower dental arches. I had never before used aluminium wire, but it turned out to have the advantage, in comparison to steel, that it could be easily shaped by hand. Only when I returned home did I learn that the Soviet Oral Surgeons used aluminium splints uniformly for the repair of their war-time trauma cases. I had a dentist's mirror and forceps, and even a few ampoules of anaesthetic solution left over. We washed the wires, forceps, pliers, etc. in alcohol, and burned them. The syringe and needle were sterilised in boiling water, and the patient received the injections. The principle is to attach a precisely fitting metal splint to the arc of the mandible, and then hold it tightly in place with metal wires placed between the teeth and around the metal splint. The upper splint must be placed first, and then the lower splint is applied, to hold the broken ends of the lower jaw precisely in place. The next step is to fix the jawbones, while the teeth are kept closed for six weeks. This rigid fixation is accomplished with thin wires.

The patient sat in front of me while I began to work in a half-sitting, half-squatting position.

The work progressed just like at home. I was delighted to be able to work, to be active in this dreadful environment where the others just sat or lay around looking grey and black, crowded on top of one another, waiting lethargically for a portion of coffee, soup or bread. Suddenly, deadly silence developed around me and, as I cautiously looked around, I noticed that an SS officer was approaching our row where we were working. His revolver case was open, but my fingers continued to twist the wires, not knowing whether he approved of our activities. Those were difficult moments while he silently passed by. A few minutes later we heard a shot and the thud of a fallen body as he stepped out of the tent. Word got round that one of the men had taken a few spoonfuls of the milk intended for some children...Including this colourful little episode, the immobilisation of the fracture took five or six hours. I received a thin slice of mouldy bread from Mrs Mayer as my reward: her husband could only consume liquids for a while. I stuffed the bread into my pocket and shared it later with Matyi, who had assisted me. Next day I checked the patient; he was free of pain, the necrosis was arrested and, a few days later, we were able to chat quietly.

After our liberation, Mayer came into contact with a German Oral Surgical Department where they examined him with only this comment: "Das hat doch ein Facharzt gemacht!" ("This was done indeed by a specialist!") They had no idea that I had learned it from their master. A few months later Mayer looked me up in my surgery at Ferenc Liszt Square in Budapest, with the request that I should replace his missing teeth with a bridge, and generally put his mouth in order, as they were emigrating to Australia.

One spring morning, I was sitting with Dr Pista Marer, an excellent specialist for internal diseases, on a little hill in Mauthausen enjoying the sunshine. We were watching about a thousand American planes moving towards Linz in a wonderful formation. We soon heard the dull rattling sounds of the exploding bombs and I turned to Pista and asked him to describe for me the symptoms of the Kala-Azar disease. He stared at me in disbelief and said: "Zoltán, are you crazy? We are on the threshold of death, with a thousand bombers overhead and you want to learn the symptoms of the Kala-Azar disease". But he told me the symptoms of this tropical disease anyway.

The ripped panel of our tent was jerked about by the wind, and we huddled together even more tightly. Someone offered vaccination cultured on Lemberg's egg against typhus, in exchange for two slices of bread. I recognised its importance, and grabbed the deal. A tall, bearded 'colleague' injected it in me. He later turned out to be a dental technician who had presented himself as a doctor, for the sake of better treatment. This made no difference to me as this shot saved my life. At the time of our liberation in Gunskirchen, both Matyi Szekely and I were suffering from the disease and, when we reached our beds in the Gymnasium Hospital in Wels, my temperature was only 37.8° Celsius - according to the wall chart - whilst Matyi's was 44°C; after suffering terribly, he died from meningitis. He had asked me for a shirt before he was transferred to another Hospital; a couple of my shirts were still in my rucksack, exactly the way I had packed them at the Ambulance Station in Budapest. The two of us were lying in our beds in the so-called 'Chief of Service' room, making plans for working together again after we got home. I felt very lonely when he left. Just before beginning my homeward journey, I went to visit the fresh new cemetery. Of the thousands of graves the guard at the gate looked up which was Matyi's. It was marked with a wooden plank. I picked some green wheat, yellow rape and red poppies from the field, tied them into a bunch and placed them next to the wooden mark on his grave.

As we were leaving for our long journey from the Ambulance Station, driven by some unexplained foresight I had packed 20 or 25 roasted coffee beans into my rucksack. At the end of our march we ate these, one at a time, to strengthen ourselves, but the coffee beans could not help our struggle against exanthematous typhus.

One day we started, abruptly, on another march. It was the end of April, the wind was blowing and it was raining unmercifully. The little houses stared at us with their doors and windows closed, as we passed through the small Austrian villages. The people in these houses must have seen hundreds of groups pass by ahead of us, yet later they could not remember seeing anything. Now it was no longer marching, but running; they herded us like animals, not with whips but with live ammunition. Irregularly, but more and more frequently we were hearing shots; whoever fell, was shot in the nape of the neck and left behind. As we were crossing one of the bridges over the River Steyr, someone said that Churchill was rumoured to have died. The reference was to Roosevelt, as we found out later, but this made little difference to us, we had been so severely cut off from news abroad, even when we were still in Budapest, that we knew virtually nothing about the activities of either one of those two. We only learned much much later about the negative rôle played by the severely ill Roosevelt at the Big Three Conference. If Churchill had not been left alone, then perhaps the fate of Hungary would have turned out to be quite different.

We were promised a wonderful new camp and, indeed, in Gunskirchen we were herded into wooden barracks which had been thrown together from still-wet logs, which were surrounded by ankle-deep mud. Just before our arrival there, we had seen some French prisoners-of-war working along the road. They yelled to us that the war wouldn't last much longer. There was a little bit of rotten straw in the area set aside for the leaders and the doctors, but the rest had only the cold and wet ground. In all, there were seven barracks with the bare ground between them, serving as latrines. Every morning, the corpses were passed through the window of each of the barracks: each could hold 2,000 people. On one of these mornings I yelled into the barracks: "Hurry up with the procedure", so that we could take them somewhere for burial or cremation, somewhere behind the camp; a German guard aimed his rifle at me and asked why there was so much noise inside, and why was I being so loud. I snapped to attention to report to him that I was a doctor and was expediting the removal of the corpses. He yelled that he had heard enough, whereupon I made an about-turn and firmly, but cautiously, began to march off through the mud, not knowing whether he was going to fire or not. That time he did not but, when one of our party failed to respond immediately to his orders regarding the removal of a body, he shot him in the head without a word. The poor boy was 17 or 18 years old.

American Red Cross parcels were distributed one day, one package between two people. Pali Koltai and I shared one like brothers, taking it in turns, enjoying that delicious condensed milk spoon by spoon. Even we began to have an inkling by that time that it might not last much longer.

The sun came out at noon one day and I stood outside the barracks to enjoy a bit of sunshine instead of the cold, wet, stale air inside, but the guard chased me back inside. Early in the afternoon I saw the same guard rushing out of the camp with two rifles, one on each shoulder. I was thinking: 'perhaps now'...but he would probably kill me... In fact, the SS Camp Commander was holding a conference with the Jewish leaders of the camp. We did not know the leaders as we were the last group to arrive. The Commander told them that he had received orders directly from Himmler to annihilate everyone by driving the camp's entire population down into a sandpit that had already been loaded with land-mines. He, the Commander, would be willing to disobey the order if the Jewish leaders would arrange for him to be issued with a pass from the approaching Americans. The leaders naturally agreed to this and set off immediately by car, flying a white flag, towards the advancing Americans. They ran into machine-gun fire - the Americans had been tricked by white flags before. In spite of this experience, they set off once again and this time succeeded in making contact. The SS Commander did receive his paper, changed into civilian clothes at once, and disappeared from sight. We were liberated! We recognised this without any emotion. They could just as well have told us that we were to be executed; we were totally exhausted both physically and emotionally.

Word came around that the warehouse had been broken open. Along with the others, I took a walk to the warehouse and returned with two 40/50 centimetre long sugar beet canes under my arms. I tossed them onto my sleeping spot and then collapsed on top of my beets and fell into a comatose sleep while clutching them. When I woke up in the morning, some groups were already leaving, but I had to rush outside to squat down because my uncontrollable diarrhoea had just begun. This was the first sign of typhus.

Later Matyi and I picked up our rucksacks and set off. We were dragging ourselves slowly along the way when, some 800 metres from our 'ex-camp' we found a gigantic food storehouse filled with sugar, American tins of meat and every kind of earthly delight. Many of the men could not resist the temptation and gorged themselves on the meat, which subsequently either killed them or made them terribly ill. We turned into a farmhouse and, totally exhausted, fell asleep in a room with two beds. We asked only for two chamber pots because we could not control the eruptions of our diarrhoea; both of them were full by dawn, but when we woke later on in the morning we found two completely clean pots next to our beds.

Our hosts were rather hospitable without being asked for anything. They seemed to be a little scared, and offered us, for lunch, some frighteningly good pork that had been retrieved from a tub of lard. Our journey continued and we arrived in Wels where we found a large Hospital already in operation. In the courtyard, Zoli Ujlaki was giving someone an injection and I decided that the place was too noisy and crowded for my taste so, as soon as I heard that a truck was about to depart for the Gymnasium (Grammar School) - where a new Hospital was to open for the sick and virtually everyone of us was sick - I signalled to Matyi and we climbed aboard the truck at once and left. Straightaway we moved into one of the rooms and named it 'The Chief Physician's Room'. Pretty soon all our companions managed to get into beds, most of them in the classrooms but those who arrived late could only find a place to lie down in the Gymnasium on the floor; at least this was not on cold and wet straw. Everyone was very weak and most had typhus. I was begging them to eat very little at a time. I found a lot of medicine in the middle of the largest Hospital room where there were some drugs to control diarrhoea, and tonics for the heart. These had most probably been put there by the Americans. We even managed to stop the most severe cases of diarrhoea with some powder containing an aluminium salt and, naturally, we tried to compensate for the loss of fluids. The same evening, a group of American physicians and medics installed one-litre size (intravenous) bottles of serum over everyone's bed, and administered them to the men. As a result of this well-intentioned intervention, a lot of them never woke up again! In time of war, if someone loses a leg, or loses a lot of blood in some other way, then serum or blood transfusion is a life-saver because the traumatised patient has a good, strong heart. The weakened, faint hearts of our companions did not have the strength to maintain the circulation against the resistance of the suddenly-increased quantity of liquid.

A few hours later the Americans arrived in the Hospital rooms with a huge sprayer and filled the rooms with clouds of DDT. When I met the commanding officer, an American Major, on the Hospital stairway, I asked him whether this powder (which was unknown to me) was effective. He ordered some lice-ridden clothing to be brought out and tossed DDT onto it. The wriggling of the lice stopped in a few minutes. The major explained to me that it was a neurotoxin and, with its help, they had been able to arrest the typhus epidemic in Naples. At the same time, he provided me with a certificate of my appointment in the Hospital, and stamped it so allowing me freely to go about even if there was a curfew.

Gradually everything became simplified and normality began to settle in. Meanwhile, poor Matyi had been taken away. A few days later the others informed me that they had spotted a little red car in a nearby garage, a car that might have belonged to the police. A few of us went over to the garage, broke into it, and I took possession of the car. My American physician colleague certified this action too. Weeks later, when the courage of the local people began to return, they appeared and officially demanded the return of the car! But I informed them that they wouldn't live long enough to witness that! I had never driven before, but one of the men had been a chauffeur in private life and he tried to teach me. I accelerated and then braked alternately - regardless of how I was going. I drove with the horn tooting at full blast, and on one occasion as I was passing a farm cart, I saw its owner kneeling down on the ground and praying with his hands together as I zipped past him. In no time at all the car had only one headlight left, had lost its bumper and the side was pushed in, but it was still running. One night, as I had to rush to the pharmacy to get some urgently needed heart tonic, an American MP stopped me with his jeep but let me go as soon as he saw my pass. Once we returned to visit the camp in Gunskirchen which stood there, deserted and silent. On another occasion, I stopped at the food warehouse and made up two packages of six tins of meat in each for Anuci, addressed them to Budapest and left them at the farmhouse where we had spent our first night after liberation. When I

87

returned a few days later to mail them, they told me that a poster had appeared announcing that all German property had to be turned in to the American authorities. There was nothing I could do about it but it really made me upset. I discovered later that Anuci had had a tremendous need for them.

The chaps were getting stronger; there were no more deaths, and life was also returning to the town. I missed Matyi though. I was alone except for the photographs of Anuci and Andris looking at me from the door of my cupboard. The season 'opened' at the swimming pool and it was interesting that every one of the young Austrian women had an English dictionary in their hands which they were studying diligently! An invisible order had appeared: *Go to bed with the American soldiers.* This order they obeyed without hesitation. So-called 'nurses' in the Hospital came up periodically and, without any discussion, stretched themselves out on the bed. Alongside the swimming pool there was a special fenced-in area, the nude bath. There was a hole in the fence and always a long queue to get a turn to take a peep. Overhead the American planes were always zigzagging and flying in, very low, over this notable area!

We were getting stronger and would have liked to get going, but this was still out of the question. I became a typhus expert and twice they asked me for consultations. Once it was for little Magda who had worked with the cooks in Koszeg. She had a very high fever although still conscious. As I lifted her shirt I saw thousands of tiny red dots. I didn't have to think much about the diagnosis. The poor soul hadn't starved as much as the rest of us and yet she was gone in a few days. Another time, a delegation from the Yugoslav camp, separated from the rest, was sent to me. They had come on behalf of a 20-year old man, quite fit, but who also had typhus. I provided them with instructions and hoped that perhaps his heart was strong enough to survive that terrible illness. As I was leaving, the leaders of the camp presented me with a red scarf. I was very touched with that and wore it all the time: I returned home wearing it.

One time, I was visiting my companions in a large ward to check their condition. The place was very neat and a German doctor was assigned to attend to them. I asked the men whether they were satisfied and was reviewing their charts when the German (or Austrian) asked me what I was doing. I said that I was checking on what was happening with my mates in the ward because I didn't trust anyone, and he was only a German and I was a Jew. He said nothing but the men told me the next day that they felt very proud of me. Many of them had known me from Koszeg.

The days and weeks were passing slowly and there was no news from home. At the beginning of July we heard that a train or two would be going towards Hungary from the vicinity of Linz. I looked up Zoli Ujlaki at his Hospital to find out whether he would come with me. We could get to the train by car. He agreed to come at once and I packed my rucksack once again. The night before, there were six vials of Penicillin among the drugs, I think the American major had given them to me as a present. I did not then know their importance. The following morning I could only find three of them. When I arrived back in Budapest, their value was well appreciated. I found my wife could replace all our broken windows from what we would have got selling those ampoules.

When I told our Commanding Major that I was returning to Hungary, he looked at me in surprise and asked why, since the Russians were there. It didn't matter, I said, after all they were my allies too. We shook hands and I thanked him for his help. As I was loading my belongings into my little red car all the men came over and gave me the addresses of their relatives so that I could notify them that they were still alive. They patted and hugged me and barely let me go. They stuck a piece of paper into my hand on which it was written in pencil that they wanted to thank me for what I had done for them, followed by many signatures; on the back they wrote: "Doctor, we saw you in Mauthausen too!" This little piece of paper is one of my greatest treasures and I still guard it with utmost care:

To our beloved Doctor

"Without sparing any effort you have fought and worked for us, to let us get our health back. You did good work, Doctor! It was successful. Please accept this humble bunch of flowers from us, as an expression of our appreciation. And we hope that soon we will be able to present to you, dear Doctor, flowers grown in Hungarian soil.

With much love,

Imre Rubin - Leo Elias - Jeno Friedman

P.S. We have read your article in the Alpenjager paper. Many of the boys from the Koszeg days will not forget what you did there, Doctor. We congratulate you."

We drove off then, with loud tooting. The horn had not shattered yet! We reached the highway and I stepped on the accelerator - we were scooting along at 100 kilometres per hour. The road was not too broad, and huge American military juggernauts were approaching from the opposite direction. Being squeezed onto the shoulder of the road, Zoli Ujlaki quietly asked, "My dear Zolti, couldn't we go a little more slowly?" An hour or two later, we reached an area where we saw some empty wagons. We stopped and parked the car on a little hill for the Wels police to find. We heard that the train was heading towards Hungary and we were trying to climb up into one of the empty wagons when a dentist colleague from Jókai Square showed up and said that he was Commander of that wagon and it was reserved for his group. We had hardly finished with the Germans and already a Jewish colleague was starting a quarrel. All the trials and tribulations had turned everyone into animals. I moved on and took over the next wagon, as its Commander. It soon filled up. After a long wait, the train finally got rolling. We travelled for many days with many stops. As we reached the Russian zone, someone called in to tell us that the commander of the wagon was responsible and would be punished unless all electrical appliances, radios, etc. were placed outside the wagon. One of the women had received a huge radio from an American soldier as a gift, and she was begging us to hide it; but I was afraid to take that chance. I became very sad when I saw all the things that had been confiscated put into a pile and burnt by the Russians. This was a little unclear and unexpected feeling.

On the journey we transferred to a Russian troop transport train, and got sunburnt in the open wagons. At Wiener-Neustadt I jumped aboard another train and then ran to the station to get some water, and bought some re-stamped Austrian stamps.

Along the way soldiers here and there tried to make a pass at one of our pretty travelling companions; we managed to frustrate their intentions even though they had rifles. Many trains, loaded with all sorts of things, passed us and hundreds of horses and cattle were herded along both sides of the railroad tracks toward Budapest. Suddenly we stopped, somewhere in Buda. I picked up my rucksack and, amidst the huge crowd, I walked over the improvised Franz Joseph Bridge. I took a tram to the vicinity of the Eastern Railroad Terminal and found a No 46 tram and then a No 10 which took me to the Ring Boulevard. I stood on one of the steps because a soldier nearly knocked me off. I got off at the Ring and walked to the Oktogon intersection where I stepped into the Brazil Espresso. Here I asked whether Anuci and Andris were alive. A nice waitress, an old acquaintance of ours, told me that she had recently bumped into Anuci. Happily I rushed on, but in the middle of Ferenc Liszt Square I had to stop and put my rucksack down, it had suddenly became unbearably heavy. I met the assistant concierge at the entrance, who told me that Anuci was upstairs in our flat. I went up in the lift and rang the bell. I rang and rang wildly but nobody opened the door. I became terrified and threw myself against the door trying unsuccessfully to break in. At last, Anuci appeared, in her nightgown and barely recognizable. She was thin, fragile, pale, but with huge, sparkling, shining eyes - she had a little cold too - and we embraced each other in silence. We had survived. I did not know then what had happened to her, but I could see that she had been through terrible times. It was the 7th of July 1945.

The very next day I began to write letters to the relatives of my mates. Of the 1800 who had left Budapest with me only 180 had survived.

It was soon after that I learned about my parents fate.

In the middle of April 1945, as the Russians approached, they were among a group ordered to go to Mauthausen. On the way, they met an SS group who drove them into a valley, shot them with machine guns and burned their bodies. The identity of the group was later confirmed by an inventory that bore Father's signature, as well as part of a dental tweezer. About a year later, we received a telephone message that our parents' remains were on their way home. We put on black suits and waited. Then one afternoon a lorry, covered with green pine wreaths and carrying their coffins, stopped outside our flat in Ferenc Liszt Square.

CHAPTER SIX

After the War
After the Liberation

(1945-1952)

In Budapest again. In a Budapest half ruined and without bridges. Together with Anuci and Andris. The reality struck us with such force that we could not believe that we had ever been separated from each other. I was reunited with Andris in Kiskunhalas where he had been staying with our maid, Margit. He waited for me at the gate and, from about five metres distance, flung himself at my neck and hung there for a long time.

So we were together at last, all three of us, and back in Ferenc Liszt Square again. My surgery remained intact. And, as if nothing at all had happened, I started to work again.

It was a strange and difficult world, to which I could not really become accustomed. Officially, it was still a democracy, with different political parties but the Communists gradually, resolutely, and without force even, grasped power for themselves. I still belonged to the so-called 'middle class', and hardly knew anything about communism. I was interested in my family and in my profession only - in the latter, wildly and passionately. On the basis of my scientific work, I shortly obtained the *Degree of Associate Professorship (Docentura) of Oral Surgery* on the 17th June 1946. The topic was: 'Surgery of the Mouth and Jaws in Practice'. I value this as the greatest scientific achievement of my life. When I presented my obligatory lecture 'The Spread of Inflammations of Dental Origin' to the Medical Faculty, to my colleagues and members of my family.

Anuci could not hold back her tears thinking of my parents who sacrificed their whole lives for this very reason and couldn't be present. I was 39 years old, and Jewish.

Once when I was walking along Rákoczi Street, I met my two old colleagues and friends of mine, Laszlo and Galocsi. We started to talk and they said: "Zolti, you have to join a party now". "Must I?" "Yes". "What kind of Party?" I asked "and to which one are you affiliated?" "We joined the Communist Party", they replied. "Too 'Red' for me", I joked, "so, if I have to I had better join the Social Democratic Party - it is more Pinkish". I could have saved myself a lot of trouble if I hadn't made a joke of it. But I was only a simple doctor.

At first, I had to go through the compulsory political screening at the Medical Trade Union and, since I had just arrived back from the concentration camps, it was just a formality.

The Medical Association, or Trade Union, after the war came entirely under Communist domination. It was, however, dictated by a man called Kaiser, a one-legged fanatic. I don't want to analyse the psychological motives of his behaviour, but it is enough to say that, in 1956, immediately after the outbreak of the Revolution, he committed suicide and died in the Hospital at Rokus.

They knew my origins, my entire life; they knew that I did not want to join the Communist Party, and in spite of all this, a female voice called me by telephone: "Comrade Frankl, would you be willing to accept the task of establishing and organising an Oral Surgical Department in the Peterfi Sandor Hospital?" Naturally, I said yes and in this way the 'regime' gave me the opportunity of developing some of the happiest professional activities of my life in a Department which dealt with the medical treatment and cure of many thousands of patients. Of course, it did not always go without a hitch, but its name shortly became well known, not only in Hungary but throughout Europe and beyond.

The liberation by the Red Army had brought great changes in the life of the country but so much hatred had been accumulated in the soul of the nation, tormented for so many decades; the fascist poison had penetrated so deeply that somebody was bound to become a scapegoat. The hatred against the victorious Soviet army erupted like a volcano. Facts and rumours spread throughout the country. The old Latin saying "Vae victis!", ("Woe to the vanquished!"), proved to be true again as so many times in history.

However, I, for my part, would gratefully kiss the hand of that tired, dirty, exhausted Soviet soldier who, just in time only some hours earlier, dropped into the Hospital where my wife and my little son were hiding in case the Hungarian Nazis should come and take them away to shoot them. The soldier got a cup of hot tea and, when dead tired, half conscious, clutching his weapon, he fell into his bed. He asked only that he should be woken up two hours later. He had to go to fight further against the murderers or perhaps to his death. This memory of that Russian soldier sank into my mind.

I started to organise my Department. We were assigned a small room which we used as a dressing room, a larger room with two dental chairs (this became the Ambulance Department) and a further room which was the Operating Theatre and painted a light blue colour. The instrument section of this Hospital was most attentive to our needs and procured all we asked for: not only those instruments needed for simple dental/surgical interventions but everything necessary for major oral/surgical operations, i.e. resection of the upper and lower jaws, treatment of fractures, transplantation, plastic surgery, hare-lip and cleft-palate operations, etc.

Slowly we trained ourselves to perform all kinds of surgery from the simple to the complicated. At first, there was a name plate outside the door: 'Dr Zoltan Frankl, Associate Professor of Oral Surgery', but, before very long, it had to be taken down on the orders of the Communist Party.

Immediately after the war in 1946 I, with my colleague Dr Jozsef Wiesner, started some research work in the Forensic Institute. It was our aim to substantiate our clinical experiences anatomically concerning the *spread of dental infections* in serious cases. Breaking through the inner surface of the lower jaw the purulent process usually makes its way towards the soft tissues which surround the gullet. From here it may spread upwards towards the cranial cavity or downwards towards the chest cavity and in most cases this leads to death. These studies were first published in the United States and were quoted in many textbooks and publications. Later, it appeared in Belgium in an International Review, complete with some new research done in an Anatomical Institute in London in 1984 ...The investigations proved that early and proper surgical intervention may save the patient's life - we have performed 212 dissections.

It was rather chilly in the large dissecting room, though the proper refrigerators were not yet working, which meant that before we could set to work we had to sweep up the mass of worms that covered the corpses. This to us was a mere bagatelle and in no way dampened our enthusiasm.

It is interesting to mention that this mortuary with its hundreds of corpses saved the lives of countless terrified persecuted persons because the heroic "Hungarian Arrow Cross" animals did not dare to enter this place.

It was terribly difficult to adapt oneself to the new society and I never totally succeeded. When I came back from the hell of the life in the concentration camp, I imagined that we were looking forward to a free and wonderful life. Being illiterate in politics we were unable to understand the events. On May 1st, 1946 in the 'Heroes Square' we listened with ecstasy to Matyas Rakosi's, the new Communist leader's address; we shouted, clapped our hands, and I even hoisted my little son onto my shoulders so that he could see our liberator better, our country's greatest man. We believed, we trusted, very naïvely, in a beautiful new world.

There were still anti-Semitic remarks being made and on the buses loud-mouthed middle-class women who could not comprehend what was going on, were fearful that they would have to return the property they had stolen from Jews. These people had, in the first days of the German occupation, denounced their neighbours and friends and even the Gestapo were startled by the fact that, within a few days, they had received messages from some 30- to 40,000 'informants'.

There were very few 'convinced' Communists, most of whom had returned from the Soviet Union, and Rakosi's first deed was to take over the so-called 'Small' members of the former Arrow Cross Party, with the aim that they might be re-educated. But it wasn't going to be easy.

For me, the difficulties started during the 'political screening' when everyone was examined to see who were the trustworthy members of the Social Democratic Party who might be forced to join the Communist Party.

In the large lecture room of the Hospital, I had to give evidence of my origins and an account of my life so far. A young, ignorant doctor, an X-ray specialist, chaired the meeting. He had previously been told that Frankl was not allowed to join the Communist Party. Today I feel ashamed that I made such a 'self-confession'.

After I had finished, Professor Erdelyi stood up and said: "Professor Frankl is not suitable to join the Party because, though he is an Oral Surgeon of European fame, he has a bourgeois mentality". When the question was put to the vote, everybody voted against my Party membership. One and all, without exception, raised their hands. When I looked around, I saw that even my closest collaborators were among them, even the young nurse whom we had started to teach.

In the Department, the practical and scientific work went on unhindered. The 'Party' however let me know on every possible occasion that I was not reliable, and continually tried to interfere with my activities. The Party Chief was a 22-year old woman whose comrades were selected from the society's lowest class and put into their position after re-education.

My chief surgery sister had once been so far to the right that, when she was travelling in a bus in Szombathely (the westernmost part of Hungary), she had actually spat at a Jew in the street - but she became an excellent Communist. In spite of this, she was able to maintain absolute discipline throughout the Department and prepared dream-like working conditions for our big surgical operations. However, she never missed an opportunity to report on me. For instance, on one occasion during a delicate operation I was starting to inject the patient when the glass syringe broke in two. As at that time it was rather difficult to obtain Penicillin, the loss was a sad one. So I lost my temper and threw the syringe to the floor shouting: "Is this the best way forward for a more effective healthcare?" - the walls in the Hospital were covered with huge Communist posters, with the text: 'Forward for a more effective healthcare'; the letters were half a metre high and written in red. The syringe was made in Hungary and I got another one and finished the treatment. After some three or four minutes I got a call from the Party Secretariat: "We have already heard about your insulting remarks in the theatre, and you will see the consequences".

The people who worked in my Department naturally followed my instructions, but the Party Members, in a covert way, always made me aware that I did not belong to them. Nevertheless we worked on and our Department became more and more famous, in spite of Communist interference.

On one occasion, the Ear, Nose & Throat (E.N.T.) Department sent a patient for consultation. This middle-aged woman was in a very grave condition. In her case, the infection had not originated from the teeth - we dealt with that problem rather often - but from the tonsils. The diagnosis was established and the patient's life was saved. Due to the gravity of the process, it was a rather tense situation when, in the middle of the examination a young girl, without knocking, entered the theatre. She stopped in front of me and, in an arrogant manner asked: "Comrade Professor, what was the profession of your father?" Being absorbed in my thoughts and having my work disturbed, I told her: "Don't you see that we are in theatre, in the middle of a very, very difficult operation. Leave the room instantly!" Shaking with anger, I tried to continue the examination and had hardly finished when, once again the telephone rang and the Party Secretary told me that it was her Deputy who had been thrown out of the room and that the matter would not be forgotten.

The Oral Surgical Department was on the mezzanine and the dental surgeries on the ground floor around the big hall. 47 dental surgeons worked there and from them we got the majority of our patients. We worked in two shifts from 8 a.m. till 2 p.m. and, next day from 2 p.m. till 8 p.m. The badly fractured lower wisdom teeth and the bleedings came, of course, usually late, at 7.30 and 7.45 p.m. This was because our colleagues strove hard to finish their work so that they could go home in time; we were left sweating and perspiring.

A kind, older man with a greyish moustache, a pensioned porter, used to stand at the Hospital gates, and once when an operation lasted so long that it was 3.30 p.m. before I started to go home, he turned calmly to me and asked with sympathetic affection: "Dear Professor, is it worth it?" I can never forget his soft, slightly sad voice. During one of the ensuing Party meetings, somebody asked whether Professor Frankl stayed so long in his Department so that he could treat his private patients!

Despite the reporting, the pestering and backbiting, our work never stopped; we loved it as we loved our patients and so the 'informers' had nothing else to report. The patients were sitting or standing in long queues in the corridor.

One afternoon, I was working in my surgery when the telephone rang. Professor Rethi, the famous E.N.T. specialist, was phoning from his surgery in the house opposite. "Dear

Colleague", he said, "don't you mind that whilst you are working, the house is burning above your head?" The concierge, the neighbours and I all ran up into the loft to find its four corners in flames. As clothes were hanging all over the loft it was obviously arson. The fire spread rapidly but, before long, the fire brigade put it out. I thanked Rethi for his warning and continued the work which I had already started.

One of the owners of the house was L. Decsi, a member of the World Champion Bridge Team and a director of a large company. A few days after the fire, I was unexpectedly called to the Party Office where, together with the Party Secretary, another woman was present. I knew she was the wife of a pharmaceutical company representative. Without any introductions they asked me about Decsi and whether I knew him. I said that we lived on the same floor, that I had treated his wife's teeth and that we had met sometimes in the past. They then started to plague me with questions: how many maid-servants did they employ? With whom did they keep company? Was it conceivable that they had started the fire deliberately so as to claim a large amount of money in insurance compensation? Suddenly I was so flustered I found I could not answer any more questions and when, in spite of their goading I was unable to give any positive answers, the woman clasped her hands together and quietly and menacingly moved her thumbs over each other and said, with meaningful emphasis: "Comrade Frankl" - not 'Zoltan' as in the past - "isn't it true that you have a little son whom you love very much?" I froze, I was unable to answer, and they then let me go. After this incident I could not take the responsibiiity of continuing my work. The Decsis later escaped to Brazil.

However, the work continued. I organised postgraduate meetings of the Hospital's Dental and Oral Surgical Departments which had achieved enormous success. At the first meeting of the Hungarian Dental Association after the war, there were only seven persons present. At our meeting when I delivered a lecture on 'The Use of Penicillin in Dental Practice', more than 120 colleagues attended, amongst them the Professor of the Stomatological Clinic and other prominent specialists. The situation can best be described as that when Dr Gollner, Assistant Professor of the Stomatological Clinic, came up in the lift with Professor Simon and Gollner asked him: "Why are these people coming here in such a throng, as if manna was to be distributed?" Professor Simon replied: "You know, my dear chap, it is real science that is dispensed here!" In our country this was the first 'summing up' of Penicillin in our profession, it was rather new to us and we couldn't yet fully appreciate its significance.

These postgraduate meetings continued for years until the Communist Medical Trade Union decided that 'organising postgraduate courses' cannot be the task of an individual but should be the duty of the newly constituted Stomatological Postgraduate Institution. The backbiting had worked successfully again. From that time on, I delivered my lectures during the regular Friday morning meetings of the Stomatological Clinic.

The practical operative surgical demonstrations were highly appraised. I performed these interventions partly in my Department, in connection with Dental Congresses, or partly in different country towns. We travelled with Elizabeth, one of my surgery nurses, to Miskolc, Kaposvar, Gyor, Pecs, Szeged, etc. and worked on the previously prepared cases for hours and hours. Dr J. Wiesner, my dearest collaborator, warned me many times: "You will burn yourself out!" Working from 8 a.m. sometimes until 11 p.m. I did not have too much time for my family.

The 3rd February 1950 was perhaps the most memorable day of my life. Some weeks before, Dr J. Kende, Director of the Stomatological Postgraduate Centre, called and told me that I was to receive a great honour, and asked whether I would be ready to see Comrade Mihaly Farkas, the Defence Minister. I told him it would be a great honour. Farkas visited my Department and told me about his complaint: his white blood cell count, normally about 6,000 in a man, jumped up for some days every month to 20-25,000 and, at such times, he felt very, very weak. He had been treated in Moscow by many eminent doctors, surgeons and dental surgeons, but they could not find the cause of his symptoms and could not cure him. Farkas, with Rákosi, had the greatest power in the county and, like him, was a callous murderer. He and his henchman's favourite amusement in the infamous prison of the Hungarian KGB-AVH was to urinate into the mouths of the already tortured or condemned prisoners. I do not know, even now, why he had been sent to me. Just as in the old days, the then Prime Minister Kallay had come to me, a Jewish Oral Surgeon, asking for help, now a Communist tyrant was desperately looking for help too, and from a politically unreliable Social Democrat.

After clinical examination, I asked for X-rays for each individual tooth and on the X-rays found only one suspicious spot. The root canal of the right upper canine was filled with gutta-percha, but the filling did not extend to the apex, and the area above the root filling seemed to be empty.

My report said that, because no other pathological factor could be traced which could have caused the damage of the blood-forming system, the possibility could not be excluded that the cause of the infection was the improperly filled empty space. I could not say with absolute certainty that this was the cause and could only prove it by operating on Comrade Farkas. After a short consultation, the attending experts unanimously accepted my opinion.

So the operation was fixed for the 3rd February 1950. Anuci was already pregnant with my daughter, Vera, and had gone into labour that morning and had to be taken by car to our friend, Professor I. Zoltan's Gynaecological Clinic, in whose care I left her. Anuci knew what was in store for me on that day as I left and hurried to the Hospital where the atmosphere was extremely restless and the Medical Officer,

Dr K. ran nervously to and fro. In my Department, however, everything was prepared beautifully, as usual. Farkas was lying on the operating table and I reassured him that nothing was going to hurt, that he wouldn't even feel the injection. He was tranquil, composed, and really confident in us.

When I lifted up the scalpel all of a sudden the door of the theatre opened softly and a head, covered with a red, flat, military cap peeped in. He was one of the heads of the Secret Police, wanting to know what was happening to his boss - it was not a reassuring moment. Simultaneously, my assistant and I looked straight at each other and we knew that, although this was a small surgical intervention, everything must be handled very carefully, otherwise we were finished. My hand stayed steady and the operation was completely successful. The symptoms never returned.

In a small adjoining room, Farkas put on his glittering uniform, and we all lined up. He said 'goodbye' to the others and then stopped in front of me and, with the comment: "Thank you, Comrade Frankl", shook my hand. I wished that he had not done so as, by ignoring our director K. the ardent Communist, in whose surgery Rákosi's portrait hung from the wall, he had bitterly offended him. We watched from the mezzanine as Farkas departed, and from the great crowd of patients in the Great Hall on the Ground Floor, 14 people, all in civil dress, stood up and followed him. They were all members of the Secret Service.

We all felt greatly relieved when he left. At 8 p.m. when I started to go home, a kind Christian colleague, gently patted my shoulder and asked: "Zoltan, why didn't you kill him?" I looked him straight in the eye and said: "How could I have done so when I was operating in the theatre?" and, physically and psychologically exhausted, I carried on with my journey.

Meanwhile, Anuci's labour was in progress. The pains became stronger and stronger and, as Professor Zoltan passed by her bed, she told him she felt as if she were lying in a liquid pool. Zoltan thereupon lifted up the sheet and, as Anuci was to tell me later, his face turned as white as snow. In a second, he had arranged for her to be taken to the theatre where he told her that a Caesarean section must be done instantly, because she had placenta previa and it was this which was causing the bleeding and impeding the birth. Before the general anaesthetic started, Anuci begged Imre that, under no circumstances should I be informed, because I was operating on Mihaly Farkas at just that exact time and, if I failed, we were finished. Anuci's operation went without any complications although, if her condition had not been diagnosed by sheer chance, it could have been fatal.

When I arrived home in the evening, the concierge Uncle Szabo told me while handing me the keys to the lift: "Congratulations Professor on your beautiful little daughter!" "What are you saying?" I answered. I couldn't believe my ears and, quickly handing back the keys, I rushed off to the Clinic. I found Anuci a little fragile, half dozing, but otherwise alright. Beside her there was a cradle and in it a round-faced little doll, called Vera. Anuci's first question was: "How did the operation go?"... and I peacefully stroked her hand.

In the Department, I had two brilliantly trained assistants and seven nurses, one in charge of the operating theatre. We had seven trolley-like operating tables with pre-sterilised and prepared instruments so that we could perform the operations both undisturbed and continuously. Relatively small operations were performed in the Outpatients' Department but usually I worked in the theatre. In this way, we could do our work more quickly and efficiently. The Hospital had 800 beds and, when it was required, we put the patients in the E.N.T. Department.

All this time I pursued very intensive scientific work in my Department.

Professor Simon dealt a lot with the local injection of anaesthetics into inflamed tissues, which he maintained were harmless. These statements started grave disputes and brought about many difficulties. I decided to get to the bottom of the question and, when I had my own Department, I ordered that all cases, including the inflamed and purulent ones, must be treated under local anaesthesia, the 2-3 and 70-80-year olds as well. This experimental 'trial' lasted for two years and it turned out that injection into inflamed tissues had no harmful effect, in fact it seemed that, in certain cases, it promoted healing. In the end, the Scientific Committee of the Hungarian Dental Association made its point of view absolutely clear in writing that this procedure, provided it was used with necessary prudence, was harmless. Professor Balogh suggested additionally that it could be combined with doses of Penicillin at the same time. After this resolution was adopted, I went home by train and, when I alighted at the Oktogon, Dr Gyorgy Istvan Fodor, one of the most famous Hungarian oral surgeons, walked up to me and offering his hand, said: "Zoltan, you have won your battle!"

However, in England, the official general direction was that local anaesthetic solutions were not allowed to be given into inflamed tissues.

On one occasion in Budapest at an official postgraduate lecture on 'The Complications of Tooth Extractions', I defended my stand on the injection of inflamed tissues. Many people contradicted me; interestingly enough, they were mainly old and anti-Semitic individuals. Then, one of the well-known Christian oral surgeons from Budapest, who was not a particular friend of mine, rushed up on to the stage and announced with deep conviction: "I do not understand why you attack Professor Frankl so vehemently, I have worked with him for some months in the same Department, and have seen him in at least 200 cases give injections into inflamed and purulent tissues, and there were never ever any harmful consequences!" He received from the audience of about 400 people, applause which lasted a full five minutes ... he had never before experienced such an ovation in his life. He deserved it because he was honest and wanted to give justice to his younger colleague who had been insulted. The lecture had started at 10 p.m. but, at 11.30 p.m., there were still 250 colleagues in the audience.

The greater part of my scientific and practical work was dedicated to the fight against cancer, i.e. pre-cancerous lesions.

The extensive surgical interventions against cancerous lesions had not given satisfactory results and it seemed reasonable that the emphasis should be placed on the *prevention* of these lesions. This was what was called 'Cancer Screening'. I drew up a paper: 'A Dentist's Guide to Diagnosis of Pre-Cancerous Lesions of the Oral Mucosa'. The paper was condensed into four pages and the Hungarian Ministry of Health sent 2,000 copies to every Hungarian dental surgeon. The result was that the number of pre-cancerous cases sent to our Department increased significantly.. This Guide was published in April 1954 and appeared in six or seven foreign languages as well. It was characteristic of its success that, in Prague in 1956, at an International Dental/Oral/Surgical Congress, I delivered a lecture on the same subject. I was surrounded by many Hungarian dental surgeons who came from that part of Northern Hungary, which had been annexed to Czechoslovakia following the Trianon Peace Treaty of 1920. One of them told me how grateful he was for the Guide and that he had stuck a copy of it on his surgery wall so that it would always be in his sight.

The thousands of successful surgical interventions, the lectures on Friday mornings in the Stomatological Clinic, the surgical demonstrations held in Budapest, and in many Oral Surgical Departments in the country, the scientific publications - all brought international fame to our Department.

During the time which was left over for myself, I had to work at home to earn money to live. The result of all this was that my family was neglected and we met mostly at meal times.

My wife also worked very hard; before the liberation, in the Hospital for Disabled Children as an Assistant Physiotherapist to Professor Zinner, the famous Orthopaedic Surgeon, and then, after 1945 in ORFI; the Institute of Rheumatology. Anuci had a healing hand; purposeful and smooth, and her stroking or bracing capacity and strengthening treatment greatly contributed to the successful healing of the patients.

We were young, and that was the decisive factor. We were young during the revolutionary transformation of the Horthy era, and even under the years of Communism. We were very fond of our families, loved our work, our friends and, despite all our hardships, we could still laugh. We were the same religion and the same age, and there was nothing of the 'stranger' between us. We discussed everything together; professional, social, psychoanalytical and political. We made excursions to the Medical House at Visegrad, to the mountains of Buda, on cheap weekend trips to the country, and rowing on the Danube ...

Our will and ambition had not been destroyed, even by the anti-Jewish laws. We had adapted ourselves to them bitterly and worked on. Anuci was always the optimist, it was she who kept up the family spirits. Like my dear father at Kiskunhalas before us, we waited, wondering whether the patients would come or not, because we too had to live. We were never rich, but we lived comfortably and we had everything we needed - meals, drinks, clothing, our children's education, theatres, cinemas, the zoo, concerts - and, above all, we had each other.

CHAPTER SEVEN

Chinese Beer and The Korean War

At the beginning of 1952, I had a telephone call from the Ministry of Health asking me if I was ready to go to North Korea with the next team of doctors, as an oral surgeon. I had no choice, it was actually an order, and anyway I had suffered a lot of humiliation and vexation at the Peterfi Hospital because I was not a Party Member. I could have saved myself a lot of trouble if I had immediately joined the Communist Party. Ever since I had been a child, I had had only one Party: that of my father who was a Royal Free Voter and Anti-Habsburg, in other words I believed in Democracy and free thought.

I accepted the mission to Korea. At that time the Red Cross groups of the other Eastern-bloc countries had already been working there. Before departure I was summoned to the Central Committee of the Party, where a lot of men dressed in black asked me whether anyone had compelled me, or had I undertaken the mission to Korea of my own free will. I answered I was going of my own free will.

I began preparations for the trip and was naturally most interested in the professional medical aspect. President Kim Il Sung had explicitly requested an oral surgeon for the village of Namri, where 147 patients with serious jaw and mouth injuries from the war awaited attention.

Extreme care was taken with our 'fitting-out'. For the cold periods we received long, fur-lined leather coats (I was travelling together with an Orthopaedic Surgeon and a Laboratory Specialist.) Apart from the fact that it was inadvisable for a non-Party man to say "No", I was really glad to have the chance to expand my experiences as an oral surgeon.

Anuci, my children, my close friends, Ibolya, Gingi, Ica and some of my Department, saw me to the airport. Two-year old little Vera put her arms around my neck and said something that sounded like "Go away!" It was only when I returned that Anuci told me that Vera had in fact said "Don't go away!"

We landed in Moscow at the Vnukovo Airport where we were met and driven to the hotel. It was a fairly long drive, and to the left the outlines of the huge university could be seen; it struck us how magnificently the city was illuminated.

Well, we were in Moscow. We received a lot of vaccinations and we had a very good time. Since Hungary had been liberated from the Nazis, we had been taught to love the Russian people and we were considered and treated as exceptional individuals. Thousands of people were queueing up outside the Lenin Mausoleum but, passing the motionless military guards of honour, we were admitted ahead of our turn. The embalmed body, in its black suit, seemed to be living, but sleeping. We visited the Kremlin, St Basil's Cathedral, with its onion-shaped domes, painted with bright, modern colours inside; the old sites where people had been executed in the past, museums, etc. One afternoon, feeling very relaxed, I had tea in the National Hotel looking onto the Square. At the department stores reserved for foreigners, we bought a pink naked plastic doll each. We must have looked odd, walking home in our thick fur coats with naked dolls in our hands. I wrote to Vera that there was a beautiful doll sitting in front of me on my writing desk (whereupon Vera told her mother: "We have a writing desk too, couldn't the doll sit there?")

The Great Theatre of Moscow was still covered with snow a metre high but people in the street were buying and eating ice creams. Among other things, we saw the Russian Ballet with Ulanova; it was indeed dreamlike. However, besides all the things of interest I had a great longing for my profession and, because it appeared that we were going to stay for a long time yet, I asked the Ministry of Health, via our Embassy, for permission to visit some Institutes and study Oral Surgery. Within two weeks I received permission to visit the teaching Hospital of Professor Yevdohimov. It was a great experience and I participated in two consultations. Upon my request, the professor's first assistant Dr Rudkov, performed an operation which I thought I might make use of in Korea. He removed a large piece of bone from a rib, to replace a missing part of the jaw. It was interesting, I learned how to do it and, in Korea, had the opportunity to perform this operation.

On one occasion, we were invited to dinner at the Hungarian Embassy. Budjonnij, the famous general of the Revolution, as well as the bespectacled Visinszkij the Foreign Minister, were present. During dinner I dropped a chicken leg on the floor and was at a loss what to do. A short podgy cook, standing behind me and seeing my embarrassment, kindly whispered into my ear: "Kick it under the table", which I hastily did. Later, he became cook at the Grand Hotel in Margaret Island, Budapest, and he always sent me delicious dishes.

At the end of April 1952 we set off again. Szverdlovsk, Omsk, Novosibirks, Irkutzk. At Irkutzk Airport there was a tiered house, the ground floor of which was for Russians only. We were led quickly through it and taken upstairs where we were offered genuine hot bortsch soup. When we arrived, the afternoon sun was shining brightly, but the following morning, the whole airport was covered with snow.

For hours we were flying over immeasurable, enormous forests. In the morning we continued our flight over Lake Baykal towards Mongolia, and landed in Ulan Bator, the capital. Ulan Bator is dominated by a main square with a huge equestrian statue, the Square being surrounded by official buildings, the theatre and our hotel. Our accommodation was comfortable, we even received toothbrushes and soap packed in cellophane. At the edge of the Square where multi-storied houses ended, sometimes the head of a camel looked at us.

Leaving Ulan Bator we headed for Peking, but suddenly landed in the middle of a desert where just one building was to be seen. There was something wrong with the engine. I could only see dozens of screws and other spare parts lying about scattered all over the place and couldn't imagine that they could ever be put back together again, but in about two hours everything was put right and we continued our flight unhindered and arrived safely in Peking where we found a comfortable hotel room and felt quite at home.

The houses in Peking were interesting, with large communal yards and rooms opening from them. The people made an extremely good impression upon us; they were industrious, hard-working, modest and smiling. Their clothes were uniform-like, blue trousers with blue jackets. There were masses of people and masses of bicycles. We had never eaten such delicious Peking Duck, but I was unable to use chopsticks. One night we were invited to the Hungarian Embassy, together with the Hungarian dance ensemble. Previously, we had thought that only the girls from the Korean dance group we had met during their tour in Hungary, were so beautiful. However, at least we could talk to these girls.

Through our Embassy, I asked the Ministry of Health whether I could deliver a lecture on my investigations relating to the spread of dental infections.

The lecture in Peking went well. I had arrived by bicycle rickshaw and spent the journey looking through my text. The Ministry had the whole text (34 pages) translated into Chinese in 24 hours. Before the lecture, there was a reception in a hall where leaders of different faculties of the university were sitting around a large table: urologists, surgeons, dental surgeons, etc.

We drank tea from beautifully decorated, transparent china cups, and discussed some medical problems. There were 200 colleagues present in the lecture room, 100 surgeons and 100 dental surgeons. Sitting on the platform were the Chairman of the meeting, the interpreter, a representative from the Hungarian Embassy, and myself. The translator was an unusually tall, very pleasant Chinese doctor, and the lecture lasted 55 minutes. I could only guess how far he had got when he mentioned the names of some of the authors I had quoted. The audience were very attentive, although one colleague did leave the lecture room. I thought to myself that perhaps he has had enough of the whole business, but he returned in five minutes. I also noticed, sitting in the sixth row, a doctor with his eyes closed and seemingly having a pleasant nap!

The lecture over and given the usual great applause, the doctor said that I was ready to answer any questions. It was then that the 'sleeping' colleague rose to his feet and began asking such difficult questions of me that I needed all my energy and concentration to answer them properly. The language of the discussion was in English and Chinese. The Hungarian Embassy representative congratulated me warmly and sincerely. All the professors mentioned above had had their education in the West, most of them having studied in the United States.

The paper was published in the Journal of the Chinese Medical Association. Much later, and just before the Hungarian Revolution, in October 1956, I was giving another lecture in Prague when a tall young-looking Chinese came up to me and asked whether I remembered him. He was my interpreter in Peking!

We took part in the May Day Parade sitting on the benches which had been set up in Tien-An-Men Square and saw, only a couple of metres above us, Mao Zedong and his escort walking up to the platform. Hundreds of thousands were marching in the procession, soldiers, athletes, and countless young children waving colourful paper flowers in their hands. Thousands of white pigeons were released into the sky and the Square echoed with singing and music.

In Peking, we were vaccinated against Japanese encephalitis, against which Chinese and Korean people had a certain immunity, for foreigners, it was 100 per cent lethal.

From Peking we travelled to Andung by train. Andung is separated from North Korea by the River Yalu. I walked down to the bank of the river and was immediately surrounded by a lot of angelic children who were extremely happy when I joined in with their games.

At nightfall, we started out by car for Korea and drove across a battered patched-up wooden and metal bridge. The winding and bumpy road weaved along woods and hills and, from time to time, we saw fireworks in the distance, followed by a thundering boom. In answer to our enquiry, our driver, a kind, friendly Hungarian boy, soothingly replied: "Oh, just a little bombardment!"

At daybreak we arrived at our post. It was a single-storied white house, standing in the middle of nowhere. Our reception was rather 'chilly' as well. Our colleagues, H. and Z. still in bed, shouted at us: "Where have you been all this time? You ought to be beaten!" They looked as if they might do it too. We were there to replace them and they were in mortal fear that we weren't coming.

Slowly we settled in, and were accommodated on the ground floor, the three of us to a single room, to await our medicines and medical equipment which were following on in another car.

We were surrounded by smiling Korean boys and girls and, in the morning, a little Korean girl would bring in warm water for us to wash.

At night, we heard strange squeaking noises coming from the ceiling; small rats were being born between the wooden slats of wood and paper. Dr L. made a rat trap in our room and caught a huge brown rat but then gave up, there were simply too many. In the same building's toilets and under our toilet seat there were numerous rats swimming about in the water just a metre from the seat and, in fear that one of these savage animals would jump up and bite them, we lifted our genitals up and protected them with our hands!

We had to be very careful about hygienic conditions. Instead of water, we were permitted only to drink *Chinese beer*. Practically all Koreans had three kinds of diseases: amoebic dysentery, malaria, and intestinal worms. There was a Hungarian girl in the group before us who had returned home with malaria. We had a charming, intelligent pharmacist, a Korean girl, who lived separately in her small hut - our pharmacy.

One day, on my way home from work, I happened to look into her room through the window and was terrified to see her lying on her bed, her face greyish-yellow, giving herself an intravenous injection. I ran into her room and asked her what she was doing. She answered, shivering, that she was giving herself Salvarsan, this being the only way to relieve her attack of malaria. By far the most appalling thing, though, was when someone was admitted with an open abdominal injury and when, at the exposure of the wound, we could see the worms (Ascaris lumbricoides) wriggling in the open abdominal cavity. Some of the worms were 10-15 centimetres long.

The Party Secretary, Comrade Borsos, received me in a rather cold manner and, the day after I met him we played a football match against the Koreans. He called me aside and said: "Comrade Frankl, you must not behave like that". All I had done was to playfully jump about in front of the opponents, pretending to frighten them! Thereafter he grasped every opportunity to be thoroughly disagreeable. It was only in my small operating room that I was 'safe' from him. He knew that I was not a Party Member or perhaps he had been instructed to keep me under particularly close scrutiny. He was about 22 to 26 years old, and the only one among us who did not work but merely wagged his tongue. He was brutal and inhuman. Everyone was afraid of him. In the event, it seemed that most of our people were on some form of spying assignment, those from the Health Authorities, the Democratic Federation of Hungarian Women, the Secret Police, and so on. Our group was a mixed bag of recruits, not a community of friends, and unfortunately for me I was still naïve.

One day, a Party meeting was called which I duly and promptly attended. I was surprised and deeply offended when Dr B. who was currently working for the Ministry of Health, whispered that I had to leave the room as I was not a Party Member. I was good enough to be sent out to the war zone, it seemed, but I couldn't participate in the 'mysterious' Party meeting.

All in all the atmosphere was very strange. Once I received a letter from home and took it, to read the much longed-for lines, to a hill some distance away from the others so as not to be disturbed by them. Our doctor/commander, J., called out to me: "Why do you separate yourself, doesn't it suit you to read your letter in our company?" It was a crime, it seemed, not to read out loud my wife's and 14-year old son Andrew's letter to me. Maybe he only wanted to show, in front of the big boss, how 'in harmony' with the Party Line he was.

The male members of the nursing and auxiliary staff spent some of their time 'womanising' and this was only to be expected, but what our Party Secretary did in his private room amounted to an orgy.

Naturally, I missed the company of women too and one afternoon I touched my assistant Kum-Szut-Ka's breasts, whereupon she drew herself quietly away and said: "It is impossible, Little Doctor. Little Doctor was 45 years old; the father of Kum-Szut-Ka was also 45 years old. Impossible", and with this, my affairs with women in Korea were over.

I proceeded to learn the Korean language. I asked the names of all objects, instruments, food and so on and, in a few weeks, could make myself understood quite well and understand what other people were saying. It was the only way to work successfully in my surgery. Generally it was hot and, since we sterilised with water, this increased the temperature of the room. Beads of perspiration kept dropping off my head and forehead, blurring my glasses during operations. I called: "Csiszti angjom!" and one of the little Korean girls on duty wiped my glasses and put them back on again for me. A barber's chair served as an operating table, and the sterile cloths, gauze, bandages and such, were supplied by Central Sterilisators. We could position the instruments properly so that everything was to hand. Light was provided by the dental lamp with a green lamp shade, which I had brought from Budapest - the same one I used in my consulting room in Ferenc Liszt Square.

The manual skill of Korean girls, the dexterity of their fingers, was magnificent and far exceeded ours. They perceived and memorised everything easily. All the same, one always had to pay attention. Normally I worked wearing light trousers and a light short-sleeved shirt, having removed my light jacket and Korean military cap. I always carried with me my small square leather bag.

The majority of patients had jaw fractures, and if the broken ends were movable and replaceable, then, after removal of the teeth and roots left between the fractured fragments, we immobilised immediately. At my station, in the village of Namri, the 147 patients had much more severe, neglected, old fractures. In such cases the broken ends moved in the wrong direction, towards the site of the fracture, and were united with soft tissue or by ossification. On other occasions there were simply smaller or larger bone deficiencies in the place where the bone had shot out. Part of these were attended to at the Centre, in the large operating room and under strict sterile circumstances. Dr J. Galambos, my surgeon friend, helped me with these operations.

I had only one Chinese patient, a boy of eighteen who was injured by a bomb splinter.

Slowly, but surely, we got used to our everyday work. The main operating theatre was in the large central building and I walked to Namri every morning, a distance of roughly one kilometre. 50 metres away from the big house, there was a rock-bunker some 14 metres deep, to which we ran when there was trouble in the sky. We didn't even know where the actual battle front was, only that it was somewhere way off from us, to the south; our only danger was from aeroplanes. We learned that, when a black dot the size of a pin head appeared in the distance, we had to run to this air raid shelter for, in seconds, that black dot would be overhead. The first few weeks passed in considerable peace, there was hardly any movement. One day, though, when the group was participating in an uninteresting 'internal' house meeting, an aeroplane droned past a few metres it seemed, over the house. Like lightning our Party Secretary jumped up and shouted: "Shelter!" and rushed out, we after him, running like mad. Suddenly he stumbled over a heap of stones and fell on his belly. All of us started to smile - this was the first uniform, harmonious action on the part of the group - but none dared to laugh out loud, we were afraid of his vengeance and of denunciation. He was the first to get to the air raid shelter. In the shelter there were two fully equipped operating rooms and an electricity generator.

At times we had Marxist/Leninist 'lessons' chaired by the Party Secretary who, in the first instance, addressed the most primitive and ignorant members present. We usually had lunch and dinner together.

From the top of the rock bunker there was a beautiful view out over the surrounding hills and forests; sometimes we sat and watched the aeroplanes away in the distance dropping their bombs.

Only a few hours distant was the capital Pyongyang and our whole group went there one day when there was a 'fair' going on. The town was rather primitive, consisting mainly of bombed-out ruins but there was a theatre - in a huge cave, some 15 to 20 metres underground. With the rest of the audience we sat on the floor and watched the performance of a war play, followed by dancing and singing. In the 'finale' the stage became full of waving red flags and there was a storm of applause.

Back at the Centre the Tetongan, quite a large river, flowed East/West to the Yellow Sea. Korean girls used to wash their linen, and we used to swim in it. We could not have been very far from the sea, as the water level between ebb and flood tides was significant. Most of the time it was hot, very hot, and on the way from Namri to the Centre by a water tap, I stripped to my waist and used to let the cool water stream down over my perspiring head and body. Thus temporarily refreshed, I worked very hard until, by the evening, I fell into bed, exhausted. I needed no sleeping tablets.

Secluded from the outside world, we worked incessantly; only the appearance of aircraft made us realise that we were at war. My little Korean helpers and my patients were very fond of me for they knew that I gave them all my knowledge and all my heart to cure them. I was happy to be among them for I could not bear the jealousy which prevailed in our group. The atmosphere was bitter, corrupted.

In the meantime, something happened that may have been insignificant, but emotionally I responded to it with great sadness. Once in Budapest in the 1940s, Anuci and I bought a round platinum Patek watch for 600 pengoes, our whole fortune. I always wore it on my wrist and - miraculously - I even managed to bring it home from the concentration camps.

Naturally, before operations I used to take it off and put it on the table. On this particular day, however, I could not find it where I had left it. I looked for it and searched for hours for it in vain. This was the only occasion when, leaning against a tree, I began crying bitterly. After all the day's work, physically and morally tired, it affected me so deeply that, although I always did my best to give and to help, I should be rewarded in this way ... I was sick at heart - so many memories clung to that watch - that even the members of the group noticed that something had happened and they started questioning me. I told them. It never came to light whether it was stolen by a Hungarian or a Korean. My depression lasted so long that - wonder of wonders - a form of solidarity arose in the group and - perhaps as instructed from Budapest - a gold Omega watch was bought for me in Peking, to replace the Patek. The Omega I wore for about 25 years afterwards, and I brought it with me when I came to England.

As time progressed, air bombardment became so frequent we were obliged to move to a shed-cum-tent next to the bunker, and here we slept together with those patients who had had operations.

Somewhere in the neighbourhood, near or far, I wasn't sure, was an anti-aircraft artillery emplacement which received direct-hit attacks every night, and every night severely injured soldiers were brought to our hospital. The saddest case was when a pregnant woman, in an advanced stage, was admitted with shrapnel having torn open her flank. She was operated on and put to bed. Unfortunately, a few hours on she went into labour and the wound reopened. Through the wound she gave birth to a dead infant and died herself, due to a haemorrhage. Soon her husband came to see what had happened to his wife and I can still hear his wolf-like howling and yelling coming from the hospital.

One morning, towards the end of August, the atmosphere became very troubled. Aircraft were flying to and fro, and the noise of the bombing could be heard everywhere. Most members of the group remained in the bunker, but I decided to go to my surgery, to Namri, as there were a lot of patients waiting for treatment. I put on my military cap and I took along my small leather bag. When I got to my workplace, the rattle of machine guns had become so frequent that, passing the house of the Korean wounded, I asked them to watch and tell me when the attack became stronger. I did not put on my gown, I just took off my coat and put my cap and bag on it. I had seen about 17 patients when the drone of the aircraft and the rattle of machine guns became so loud that I felt I had to go 'home'. I took my cap, my coat, my leather bag and hurried off. The Korean soldiers, looking out through their window, were giggling as they saw me. Apparently they had had more experience in similar attacks.

At first I couldn't make up my mind which way to go. To the Camp? i.e. to the bunker, I would have to cross a small forest divided into two by a white highway. Thinking that this route would be clearly visible from the sky, I continued my way to the left, into the wood where the Koreans had an open bunker. Actually, it was a plain walled pit dug out from the ground and measuring four by six by three metres deep. I reached it and found already sitting there the Korean officers and, among them, the little pharmacist girl. So I slid down to them and settled down against the shorter wall of the hole and, driven by some unforeseen impulse, put my hard leather bag over my head. It turned out later that that was what saved my life.

Theoretically my idea of avoiding the highway proved to be right. A Korean nurse who elected to go this way, was hit by machine-gun fire in the thigh, which broke the bone and she died shortly after from the injury.

Our driver, unfortunately for him, decided to take his normal route to Peking in spite of the bombing. His car passed our bunker some 15 metres away and, as the car was an easy target as seen from above, a bomb hit or fell in his immediate vicinity. He was thrown out of the car but a large piece of mortar fell into the renal part of his body and he was severely injured. I felt a terrific explosion, my vertebral column, leaning against the earthen wall, was frightfully shaken and then the earth fell over on top of me and I was sitting paralysed. My leather case had saved my head from direct injury and as I carefully tried to move my fingers I realised that they hadn't become paralysed. Otherwise, completely buried I could not move and then I heard the little pharmacist scream: "Dr Frankl!" after which I was dug out. I saw the little girl taking off her pullover, perhaps in order to cover me, then I spat the dust out of my mouth which was full of blood. Two Koreans looked at each other thinking that I must have a lung injury, but I knew that I had just bitten my tongue. I do not remember how I was pulled out of the pit, I only know that, supported by two men with long, uncertain strides as if I had become paralytic, we ran towards the Centre. Half flying in the air, I kept shouting: "I want to go home, I want to go home!" The rest is a little obscure. I was carried into a room, undressed, and my vertebral column was tapped to see if there were any fractures, then I was put to bed.

When I came round, I felt a horrible pain in my back, along the vertebral column. I was given Codeine to relieve the pain, but it only helped for four to five hours. I suffered in agony, groaned and wriggled incessantly. The moaning disturbed my colleagues to such an extent that they put my bed outside the tent. From there at night, I crept stealthily, with faltering steps, to the small table where the medicaments were kept, to get some Codeine for myself.

My Korean patients had great compassion for me. A little girl with blue underpants used to sit at my bedside for hours, but she could not relieve my pain. The blue pants I had brought from Budapest. During an operation at which she was assisting there was massive bleeding and her skirt and underclothes were covered in blood so I had to replace them.

Meanwhile, my ears too began to ache and my colleague, Dr S., established that both my ear drums had burst and that I already had a middle-ear inflammation.

Then, one day, it was decided - surely on instructions from Budapest - that I was to be sent home. I packed my case histories, my models, my X-rays, photos, my diary and, before leaving, I went to the Party Secretary's room where I found some black coffee which I quickly gulped down before going out of the house where my Korean patients were lining up to say 'good-bye'. I went from one to the other and, calling each of them by their name, I shook hands with all of them, taking my leave. I was greatly surprised, though, that my theatre nurse whom I had worked with for months, was not among them. I was put on a lorry and the journey, the most horrible journey of my life, began. My injured spinal cord was cruelly shaken on the long, uneven road. There was no rest, only pain. The Party Secretary came with us. On one occasion they made me stand up so that I could urinate from the edge of the lorry. On another, I had to drag myself off the lorry and seek shelter under a bridge because there were so many aeroplanes overhead.

From the border town of Andung I went by train to Peking in the company of our injured driver, lying next to each other on a board placed on top of a passenger carriage. Incessant Chinese music came from an extension speaker and that irritated us so much, but somehow we managed to switch it off.

At Ferihegy Airport in Budapest I was met by Anuci and Dr R. I must have been very pale for Anuci immediately told me to put my luggage down. We embraced each other and I was taken to the hospital in Kutvölgyi Road, where I had once been taken in a 'closed' car for a consultation with Rákosi's brother.

I was allowed two visitors only; one was naturally Anuci and the other I chose to be my sister-in-law Ibolya. At first I thought of my brother Sanyi, but they were so indifferent to Anuci during my absence that we became rather distant from each other. In the Hospital they tried everything on me. A young oto-rhino-laryngologist examined my ears and said they would never recover. But, one day, my old friend Professor Gy. V. happened to come into my room and asked me what I was doing there. I told him about my ears, he examined them and said that these kinds of war injuries always heal! And so it turned out.

After about a fortnight, the Director of the Hospital came into my room accompanied by the then Minister of Health, Dr Doleschall, who proceeded to ask the Director what information had been heard concerning Comrade Frankl's injury The Director answered that, according to rumours, Frankl returned home in a night-shirt. Whereupon Doleschall remarked that, under the circumstances, it was going to be difficult to get a replacement. Then, turning to me, *he asked if I would be willing to state that I had been injured due to my own fault! I categorically refused - we had already heard of the 'self-confessions'.* It was finally agreed that I had fallen out of a car and that was the reason for my injury. As if nobody knew that there was a war going on in Korea.

For a long time my backache persisted and, one after another letters from Korea were delivered, letters decorated with coloured drawings, bearing messages of love and wishing me a speedy recovery.

When I visited my Department I found, on my operating table, a beautiful bunch of white lilies surrounded by green leaves. My theatre nurse had put them there.

During working hours one morning, I was suddenly overwhelmed with terrible pain and was obliged to go and lie down in our small cloakroom. The 'spies' got to work and, in a few minutes, Dr Gy. K. arrived and barked at me "How dare you lie down in working hours".

All this happened because, at the festival dinner party where medals were awarded to members of the Group, a great injustice was inflicted upon me. The awards were distributed by A. Ratko, Minister of Health. I had naively supposed that, in addition to the first prize, the gold medal, I was also going to receive an additional decoration as well because I had been wounded while fulfilling my duties. To my great surprise, gold medals were distributed one after the other, but I was only given a bronze medal, the same as awarded to the orderly of the Pathologic Laboratory at St. Rokus Hospital. In other words, the Consultant, the Associate Professor of Oral Surgery and the orderly were on the same level! At first, I was inclined to refuse it and remained seated, though I knew that finally I *would* have to accept if I was to avoid getting into trouble, as Stalin and Rákosi were still in power.

The disadvantage of my 'award' was more or less felt by all in the Hospital too and yet, later, I was elected to the Presidium of the Patriotic Popular Front. At the start of the Imre Nagy era, I was even asked by them to deliver a lecture to a large audience in the Hungarian Theatre. I pointed out how many mothers and infants had died in Korea as a consequence of the American bombing attacks. A few weeks later the 'Black Voice' of the "Szabad Europa Radio" station broadcast that Dr Zoltán Frankl, Chief Oral Surgeon at Peterfi Sandor Street Hospital always asked his patients whether they were Communists because, otherwise he would not treat them. "Radio Free Europe" in Munich told such lies, just as later, during the Hungarian Revolution in 1956 when it kept howling: "Fight boys, do not stop, our planes are on their way!" - and the 'boys' were lying in wait on the rooftops for the much promised aeroplanes from the West, but the planes never came. Afterwards, the whole staff of Radio Free Europe were relieved of their office.

The reason or motive for my 'award' was as follows: on behalf of the Party, the Group Secretary was in charge of our well-being and should have returned the Group intact.

However, because he failed to fulfil his task, he tried to put the blame on me. He stated that I was not careful enough, that I was looking for danger. He being a Party Member and me not, naturally they accepted his version of the story. In the event, this insult largely contributed to my leaving the country later.

Looking back at my time in Korea - a communist country - I am very struck by one fact: due to my experience in treating some rather unusual cases of war injuries, I invented a new method of operation and wrote a thesis about it. This paper about the treatment of jaw injuries was published in the *British Journal of Oral Surgery*, in a capitalist country, in 1968. Another work of mine 'Plastic Surgery for Reconstruction of Seriously Injured Soft Tissues' was delivered in a paper at an International Congress in Aosta, Italy, in 1975. These two examples show that in the science of medicine there is no 'Iron Curtain' between Communist and Capitalist countries. The aim is sacrosanct: to treat ill, or injured people in the best possible way, irrespective of any politics.

CHAPTER EIGHT

The Hungarian Revolution

The 23rd October 1956 started just like any other weekday. I worked in the afternoon shift from 2 pm till 8 pm. We worked hard, particularly after 7 pm, for this was the time when our dentist colleagues used to send upstairs (the Oral Surgery being on the mezzanine floor) the most carelessly fractured, lacerated, deeply broken roots, because they were in a hurry to get home as early as possible.

Wearily, I went downstairs. Fortunately, outside the Hospital, there was a taxi-cab and I headed for it. The driver was a woman. Before getting in, it struck me that there were many more people than usual hurrying from Rottenbiller Street towards Rakoczi Street. I asked the driver what was happening. "Where are all these people heading?" "They are going to take over the Radio", she replied. The Revolution had begun. Silent and weary I got into the cab and we drove home to Ferenc Liszt Square.

Arriving at our flat on the third floor I found no one at home except for Vera, who was then six years old, and our maid. I walked up and down in my room while, from downstairs, I heard shouting and distant sounds of gun-shots. Suddenly the telephone rang - it was Andris, now 18 years old. "What are you doing? Where are you?" I asked, on tenterhooks. "I'm helping to demolish the statue of Stalin". "Don't you demolish anything", I said. "Come home immediately!"

Now it was Anuci only who was missing, and she rang about half-an-hour later from the house of a friend of mine, Michael Gerendas, Leader of the National Blood Centre, who lived near the Central University in the vicinity of Museum

Boulevard. It turned out that she had been present at a meeting of the Petöfi Circle where my colleagues, as pale as death, had been listening to the charge brought against them, for the actions they had committed during the Stalin/Rákosi era. They knew very well that these charges were true. Leaving the extremely 'excited' meeting, they had heard shots from the direction of the Radio building, and then Anuci had gone to the Gerendas family's flat. When it became a little calmer outside, though shots could still be heard, Mike escorted Anuci into the street and helped her to get a taxi to take her home. She was very excited, entirely under the influence of the meeting, but we were happy to be all together at last, and at home.

Although I didn't say anything to anybody about it, I was convinced from the first that the Revolution could not succeed. After the disastrous Treaty of Yalta, the gigantic Soviet Union with its huge armed forces was ready to protect its satellite, and the highly indoctrinated and servile Hungarian government. It turned out that the initial purpose of the Revolution had been a purely *nationalist insurrection* against a foreign, occupying power and its servants. Alas, later, other elements surfaced as well. Within a few days a Jew was hanged in a town called Miskolc.

The first speech of Archbishop Mindszenty, Primate of Hungary, after the outbreak of the Revolution, remains forever in my memory. According to Mindszenty, who was to become a martyr and idolised by the West, the first and most important task was to return the ecclesiastical property confiscated by the Communist Government immediately to the church. The Hungarian youth had fought for *Liberty*, not for church property; they did not even want to overthrow the Socialist system, but wanted to decide on the future of their country for themselves.

The following day I went to work again, as usual. There were a huge number of people moving about in the Hospital lounge and leaning over the banister - my assistant D.K. and I

127

were watching them. K, quietly remarked: "It's beginning now", for we had once agreed that, if he were informed of a change in the regime, he would warn me. He was a firm rightist but in 'hard' times he served me faithfully and was a marvellous surgeon. After the suppression of the Revolution he became most arrogant, ungrateful and malevolent. I responded very carefully for I already knew that I was soon going to leave the country and I would have nothing to do with such people.

Soon the wounded began to arrive. Someone came running from the E.N.T. Department: "Professor, hurry up, come quickly, a patient is bleeding to death!" I ran upstairs and saw a middle-aged man sitting on a chair. Blood was shooting out from below his jaw. We carried him gently downstairs to my operating room and laid him on the table. A bullet had entered below the right lower jaw, passed through the floor of the mouth, broken the jaw and had left through the mouth. Ligating the bleeding artery of the tongue we cleaned the wound then, removing the fractured teeth, we splinted the broken jaw. Others came, some on foot, some on stretchers. There were some who begged me not to put their names on the records - or used false names.

One of my most exhilarating cases was when an extremely handsome young man was lifted onto the operating table from a stretcher. He was a fine, strapping lad, so tall that the table was hardly big enough for him. In his huge grey/green eyes there was deadly terror like that of a hunted animal. Stroking his head, I said to him: "Don't be afraid, my son, nothing harmful can happen to anybody here, and you won't feel any pain". There were several young men in the operating room and one of them tapped me carefully on the back and whispered: "Professor, he is a State Security man!" I raised my head and, in the deadly silence, declared: "In my operating room there are no State Security men and no Revolutionaries, there are only patients and injured people!"

128

I operated on the boy immediately; he only had a slight injury to the soft parts of his face, caused by a bullet and, within a few days he was healed. I heard afterwards that, when he had been put outside the theatre to make way for another patient, one of the boys had bent over him and said: "We are going to finish you off". Meanwhile, the machine-guns kept rattling, uninterrupted, on the roof of the house opposite. Slowly we got used to them and went on working incessantly, even after the Russian invasion on the 4th of November.

At home, of course, there was no peace, for Andris, a medical student and member of the University-Brigade, was in the thick of the fighting. He and his fellow fighters were sitting behind their machine-guns and, about 200 metres away, dozens of huge Soviet tanks were lining up. Luckily they had received instructions from the Central University not to shoot. When everything was over, they wrapped their guns and ammunition in sheets and buried them in the garden of the neighbouring Institute of Anatomy. The trouble was that, when later the guns were found, the sheets bore the mark in red letters: '2nd Gynaecological Clinic'. The rest I only know from hearsay.

The boys tried to run away; one was hanged and several of them imprisoned. Andris was not among them, he was seriously ill with erysipelas and lay in bed in the Clinic basement. The first person who dared to go and see him was Frici, Anuci's brother. Then, the day after, I brought Andris home in a van as his life was in danger in the Clinic.

In December a young man from Sopron helped Andris over the Austrian frontier for money. By a quirk of fate a few weeks later the same man came to see me at my Department asking me if I knew some way for *him* to defect to Austria too. Of course I couldn't help. He got the second part of the agreed amount only when he had handed me Andris's handwritten letter saying that he had got to Austria safely. I was just giving an injection to a disabled patient who, for some reason or another, had a lock-jaw and so was sent to me. I had finished the injection but then began to feel faint. All I could do was to ask my colleagues to perform the necessary intervention, and I staggered into our small dressing-room and dropped onto the couch.

Three doctors were called in to examine me, but they were unable to find out what was wrong. Two of the nurses offered to take me home but, on the stairs, I felt giddy again. Once more I was examined by a woman colleague, but all I remembered was sitting at home in one of our armchairs feeling dizzy.

I did not want to lose my son, and I did not want to leave Hungary. But if I had to choose, the safety of my family came first.

Meanwhile the fighting went on. It was not the first, nor the last lie of the Voice of America Radio Station when it called upon the youth of Hungary to continue the fight, saying that their aeroplanes were on the way. The children were watching and waiting on the roofs for the aeroplanes from the West that never arrived. At the corner of Ulloi Road and Ferenc Boulevard, a Soviet soldier was flattened as thin as paper by Russian tanks rumbling over him and at the corner of Andrassy Road and Terez Boulevard, a State Security man was hung by his feet from a tree. Soviet tanks, turning their conning towers right and left, were dashing along and shooting incessantly. Through one of the windows in Jokai Square, two elderly sisters were looking out; in a moment they were both riddled with bullets.

At the Department the work continued. After the failure of the Revolution, I used to walk to the Hospital between Soviet tanks lining the streets. There were no trams or buses and there wasn't even room for a bicycle. One night, at about 10 o'clock, I was on my way to a patient when, in a deserted street, a Soviet soldier approached me, but when I said: "Vracs" (Doctor) to him in Russian, he went peacefully away.

On the other hand, one of our neighbours went out into the street, having been informed that bread was being distributed in the neighbourhood. He never tasted that bread; a bullet killed him instantaneously.

My diary at this point gets confused like the events they record. On November 4th, muffled explosions woke me up and I rang Police Headquarters to find out what they were. "A small attack, Professor", was the answer. The invasion had begun.

Hundreds were killed, thousands interned and many thousands taken to the Soviet Union. I knew nothing for certain as, at that time, I just went on working.

And then the country began to swarm with people trying to flee - by train, by car, by bicycle, or on foot - and, within a few weeks, about 200,000 people had left the country for the West.

Andris's girlfriend, pretty little Zsuzsi, who lived across our street in Ferenc Liszt Square (Anuci used to stand outside waiting for Andris to come or leave, during the troubles) came over one night to say 'Goodbye' to us. In the hallway she said to Anuci: "I love Andris dearly". They met once again in Vienna in December, then she went to Maine in the USA, and Andris to England.

Anuci, Vera and I followed Andris on the 22nd May 1957.

CHAPTER NINE

Emigration and Epilogue

After the Hungarian Revolution was crushed, Anuci set about in earnest to organise the plan for us to emigrate. Her request for a passport and visa had been sent months before to the proper authorities, as she wanted to visit a childhood friend in London. Her trip was authorised and, interestingly, her passport was stamped on 23rd October 1956 ... the first day of the outbreak of the Revolution. I, for my part, had had an invitation to an International Oral Surgical Congress in Venice, for May 24th 1957. I wrote immediately to the Congress Chairman, Professor Saraval, asking him to send me another invitation and, at the bottom of the letter, I put a note: 'Periculum in mora!' (Danger in delay!). This warning in Latin was usually put on medical prescriptions only in emergency cases, so that the pharmacist should disregard all other prescriptions and deliver, instantly, the one in question. The new invitation arrived by return of post.

Actually, I did not want to emigrate. Despite all, this was my homeland. My father had brought me up to be a true Hungarian. I had brought up my family in Hungary, building up my professional and scientific life, and Hungarian was my mother tongue. I could read in German and English but I could not speak English.

A man who is *fifty years old* or more should never try to emigrate. He should not leave his homeland because his roots are very deep and what he loses he will never find again. Only the children are worthy of the sacrifice; they are young, they can start a new life, they will be happy even if they are sometimes drawn back by a form of nostalgia to the abandoned home of their parents.

In Hungary, everyone had an identity card and, when travelling abroad, this 'card' had to be deposited at the nearest police station. After Anuci had arranged to add our daughter Vera's name to her passport, she deposited it at the 6th District Police Station. My journey was authorised by the Ministry of Health and therefore my passport was deposited there. Since at that time married couples were not allowed to leave the country together, this was the only way for us both to leave at the same time. My medical books were sent earlier to Andrew (he had now taken the English version of his name) in London and he had received them, but otherwise we left hurriedly and completely financially unprepared.

On a damp, grey morning two trains were standing next to each other and both ready for departure. The first was going to Vienna, the other towards the Yugoslavian border and Ljublana. Some of our friends were standing there in the half light. The train to Vienna departed first: Anuci and Vera were on it. As their train began slowly to move away, little Vera lifted her arm to wave a farewell. My train departed seven minutes later.

On the Hungarian side of the border they did not bother me, but the other man in my compartment was taken off the train and, in the station building, he even had the heels of his shoes searched. When we arrived in Ljublana we had quite a lot of time to spare and I went to look around the town. It was a depressing experience; the streets were dark, unfriendly and deserted, so I returned quickly to my carriage.

Early morning in Trieste - and the contrast was colossal. Everything was sparkling in the sunshine. There was a bustle of work and a new, bright, colourful world unfolded. In Venice, at the station, a great number of people were milling about. I only knew one person in the town: Professor Saraval. I went first to his surgery and from there to a third-rate hotel 'The Budapest', run by expatriate Hungarians. We had left Hungary on May 22nd; I arrived in Trieste on the 23rd and, on the 24th, I delivered my lecture, in Italian, to the Congress in Venice. Meanwhile Anuci and Vera had arrived in Austria, and a couple of days later they arrived in England.

I had received a visa for England in Hungary but, when I went to the British Embassy in Venice, I was told that this visa was not valid from Italy. The situation was rather awkward because I only had thirty dollars, the maximum allowance from Hungary. So I applied for a new visa. It took three months to arrive.

Once, while walking on the street an elegant gentleman came from the opposite direction and addressed me suddenly, greatly surprised. "Zolti, com' va?!" ("How are you, and where are you going?!") It was Bruno Jarach, the husband of a woman I had once treated in Budapest. It had been 22 years since I had last seen him in that city. He had seen me only once in his life but he still recognised me there in Venice. He became acquainted with my financial situation and, from that time on, he supported me regularly.

While waiting, I got to know Venice, the Doge's Palace, the Church of Frari with the tomb of Canova, and Titian's wonderful painting of Madonna Assunta. I walked up and down the Piazza San Marco and always drank my espresso in the same café. I 'phoned Anuci occasionally, who reassured me that I should wait patiently, that the visa would arrive. I cruised over to the Lido with a vaporetto, lolled about in the soft, white sand, and swam a lot. I often used to visit Professor Saraval's Oral Surgical Department and went with him to Teatro Fenice for an English Theatrical Company's performance. He assured me beforehand that I would not understand one single word. It was Shakespeare's play *Titus Andronicus* and, to our great surprise, we understood every word, perhaps because Laurence Olivier played the main role. Once I had enough money to travel to Lake Garda and Gardone and took a steamer to its upper end Riva.

At long last, the visa arrived and on the evening before my departure I was invited to dinner at Saraval's. He had a beautiful wife. Next day they saw me out to the airport and Bruno provided £20 for the fare.

The aeroplane started from Venice at nightfall and Anuci, with Vera, whom I had of course phoned ahead, set off in good time for Heathrow Airport. They waited and waited but there was no sign of the aircraft. Enquiring about it they were told not to worry, as Italian aircraft never signalled ahead, but ultimately they always arrived! When I alighted from the plane, I saw a long, black shadow waving from the observation tower and heard the familiar whistling. It was my son Andrew, who at the time was working as a waiter at Lyndhurst in Hampshire and had just arrived at Heathrow at the last minute. The family was united again: Anuci, Andrew, Vera and me.

But soon after my arrival I fell into a deep depression. Around me I felt, was nothing but thin air. Leaving behind my country, my Department, which I had built up with so much love and care, losing our flat, my surgery, being separated from my friends.

I didn't want to come away, as a Hungarian poet once said. "I was swept away, like a leaf, by a *whirlwind* ..." Swept away by the hurricane of history like the other 200,000.

At least in England I was not the 'Jew' and they did not make me conscious of being one. I was not called *bourgeois* or asked to which Party I belonged. I was just a foreigner.

My wife Anuci, on the other hand, was extremely happy, and my children Andrew and Vera, through hard work, built up a happy and harmonious lifestyle. Andrew gave up Dentistry after the first year and graduated in Economics at the University of Sheffield and started to work at the Ford factory in Dagenham. Later, he established himself as the co-proprietor and publisher of the highly successful 'Car' magazine. Andrew also organized popular Truck Races. He had charm, good manners, and modesty. He kept his

Hungarian connections and became the English correspondent of the Hungarian paper *'Automotor'*.

My daughter, Vera, got her degree in History at Warwick University and then devoted herself to journalism, having articles and reports published everywhere in the world. After several years at the BBC World Service, she now works mainly with English, American and Canadian Broadcasting Companies, and is the regular correspondent of National Public Radio in Washington. She is pretty, clever and talented. Her boyfriend, Etienne Duval, is also a journalist - his mother is Scottish, his father French, and he is a very, very charming man.

Andrew married June, an English girl, and they had twins, a boy and a girl - Nicholas being 27 minutes the elder. Nicholas is interested in mechanics, electronics, and computers; he is not fond of reading and writing. He is excellent at all sports, rugby, tennis, cricket, skiing, swimming and so forth; whereas his sister, Annabelle, is much nearer to classical studies and is an expert dog breeder, thus following in her mother's footsteps. She adores riding, particularly her own horse, Dylon. Annabelle is also an excellent sportswoman.

Well, I was here in England, but not the same man as before. I couldn't see clearly, and even now, as I write about it, I am hazy about what happened next. I seemed to lose my strength. The sharp memory, the intellectual capacity to react, disappeared. The talent to observe and to debate firmly, so much admired by my friends and feared by my scientific adversaries, hardly existed anymore. My willpower which until then had carried me through all the hellish difficulties of my life, seemed to have run out. Instead of being like my wife and children, and starting out cheerfully on this new life, I was overcome by an unexplained lack of vitality. I was tired, I was kept back by the past. This sad condition, so different from any other illness, lasted a long time. Andrew told me that I would be able to earn my living, but that I would have to forget my scientific ambitions.

Our particulars were registered in some office or another and I informed them immediately that I had been ordered, as an Oral Surgeon, to North Korea, but was not, and never had been a member of the Communist Party.

I thought that life would now continue smoothly, but it turned out that, despite my Hungarian degrees, I had to take the so-called Statutory Examinations before I was allowed to practice. It sapped my remaining strength since, in Budapest, I had been the examiner and now, here, I had to become a student again! Those refugees who were not doctors or dental surgeons or lawyers were in a much better position; they were able to start to earn money immediately. Before the examinations, we had to visit and work in a teaching hospital. I was posted to the Royal Dental Hospital for six months, with one of my right-wing colleagues. Unfortunately I was posted to the orthodontic and children's departments, even though I did not like either.

Apart from all this, I was concerned with another personal matter. In Graz, Austria - one of my wife's uncles was married to a rather unhinged woman who had once taken a pot shot at her husband. For some reason she had got angry with us and reported me to the Home Office and MI5, informing them that I was a notorious Communist spy. My wife and I were summoned to the Foreign Office in Whitehall and duly arrived with our passports. We had to go back many times. I was interrogated by a civil servant who asked in which room my passport had been issued in Budapest and where had I to put the necessary 'mark' permitting me to leave the country. He wanted to know, if the need arose, would it be possible to 'bring somebody out' from Hungary? Of course we did not have the faintest idea what it was all about, who had denounced us, or of what we were accused. And then, by a lucky accident, Frici, Anuci's brother, sent us a letter written in German to him from the above-mentioned woman in Graz.

In the letter she explained to Frici that she was now able to ruin the Frankls in London. Apparently, after the war, a detachment from the British Secret Service had stayed in their castle in Wies. She had become friendly with them, and she wrote them a letter denouncing us. It was pure fabrication, of course. The next time we were called to Whitehall, we handed over this letter and at once the attitude of our interrogator changed. At long last he could see the situation clearly; he thanked us and let us go once and for all. The whole affair seems very simple now, but at the time it was very worrying, as we did not see how it would end. It didn't have a beneficial effect on my depression either.

English people were on the whole phenomenally gentle and nice to the Hungarian refugees. It is typical of their character that they try to help the 'down and outs' with warmth and affection. This was especially true after the crushing of the Hungarian Revolution. Special committees and institutions were established and money and clothes were collected. The British Council for Aid to Hungarian Refugees helped us as well, and gave us money monthly for food and lodging. We rented a two-roomed flat at 24 Belsize Park Gardens, in Hampstead, London, where so many refugees lived, mainly German. There was even a story going round that when Churchill announced in the House of Commons "we have won the war" - he added: "however, Hampstead is still not ours!"

Vera was at this time 6½ years' old and had to continue her studies, so Anuci went around Hampstead to find a school. Strolling from street to street she caught sight of a plaque on a house: 'School for Girls'. She went in and said that she had just come from Hungary and had a daughter for whom she would like to find a school, and would they be able to help? She was told in a straight and simple way that she could bring in her little daughter, because they thought their school would be very suitable for her. Anuci did not ask any financial questions; in Budapest one did not have to pay for school. Vera went regularly to school and they became very fond of her. One of the teachers, Stevie, took her under her wing and taught her proper English. For instance, Stevie would say "Umbrella", and simultaneously draw one. Vera dutifully repeated words, one after another, and in this way, her English became perfect. Anuci was told only much, much later, that St Christopher's School was a very expensive private school, but when she went shamefacedly to explain, no fees were accepted from her. She was told that, when her husband had finished his Statutory Examinations and started to earn some money then, and only then, should she come to pay. And, when she did go back to pay, the amount they accepted was ridiculously small.

My colleagues at the Dental Hospital received me with kindness and understanding. They saw this queer fish, this foreign professor walking around sadly, head bowed down, minus his Department and without his country. I sat down to eat with the consultants and the students and was very much disturbed that my English wasn't good enough. They helped me in the Department because I was not very good in Orthodontics. Professor Walther and Mr J. Hovell were very charming and lenient. But, it seemed, I still remained a 'foreigner': When it had become apparent that someone had accepted a pound note from a patient, I was the one who was asked "Was it you?" However, I did not notice any anti-Semitism from anybody and I continued my work taking impressions, making fillings and so forth.

The time of the Examination was approaching, which filled me with terror.

On the great day I started off early one morning in the direction of Hampstead Underground Station. We had to carry our hand instruments in a wooden box, and I can see before me now the weary depressed man that I had become. Somehow I arrived at the Hospital. We had to take impressions with Alginate material from the upper and lower jaw of a patient, and set in two wax bites. The patients were sent for and paid. Unfortunately, I had made holes on the trays to ensure better fixing of the material. The result was that, when I took the impression, the material went through the holes so that, in the end, only the tray was visible. I cleaned the tray and started to mix the material again, but the rubber cup fell out of my hand and I had no time to take a new lower impression. The upper was good and so was the wax bite, but the lower tray remained empty. Only one thought went on in my head, round and round: "I won't pass! I won't pass!" and I didn't. When Anuci and a colleague took me home by taxi I started sobbing. The news that the Hungarian professor failed to pass the examination spread with lightning speed. Officially I should have left the Hospital, but Professor Pickard somehow arranged for me to stay on.

In 1985, when the American Endodontic Society elected me Honorary Fellow and the British Dental Journal even published my photograph, Pickard wrote a wonderful letter of congratulations. To this I replied that this honour was, in reality, due to him as, without his help, I could never have achieved it. At the next opportunity I passed both the first and second parts of the examination. But the bitter memory of this grim episode haunted me for a long time.

The drawback was that the other Hungarian Dental Surgeons had already started their practices whilst I was still finishing my Examination. One of them who had a good business sense, circulated throughout the camp where they were billeted when they arrived in England, a printed note with the inscription: 'K.Sz. the Dental Surgeon of the Hungarians'. I did not know where I should start, but my family insisted that, because of my qualifications, I could only start in Harley Street, one of the most famous medical districts of the world. And so it happened. I started to work on the 31st August 1958, in my surgery at No 7 Upper Harley Street, and I have worked there ever since.

After I finished the Statutory Examination in 1958, I immediately joined The British Dental Association. Later I became Chairman of the Northern Section of the Metropolitan Branch of the British Dental Association between 1966 and 1969. However, I performed my most intensive scientific activity at the Anglo-Continental Dental Society from 1958. I organized and became Chairman of its Study Group for 25 years and its President from 1977 to 1980.

In short, my practice had started. First came the Hungarians, some of whom I had already treated or operated on in Hungary. I saw again the crowns, bridges and fillings, which had been made 20 years ago, settled and unchanged in the mouth. One recommended me to the other. Then came the patients from England, from abroad - Americans, Canadians, Germans, Italians, Indians, Chinese and Africans. Among them was the King of Ashanti (Ghana). He was highly cultured with degrees from Oxford and Cambridge; he would wanted to take my wife along to become his fifth wife - but Anuci somehow did not want to leave me! I was a little apprehensive when one of Patrice Lumumba's bodyguards came for an extraction. He was so tall that he had to duck his head when he came through the door, and that was more than two metres high, but his tooth was extracted smoothly, without any pain.

The '60s were the decade of countless lectures abroad and holidays in England and overseas. The most significant among these was my first meeting with Professor M. Bouyssou of Toulouse University, who asked me to join the Groupement International pour la Recherche Scientifique en Stomatologie. Until his death in 1984 he was my dearest colleague and mentor. We worked together in many scientific areas, his photograph is on the wall opposite me, and his wonderful English with its characteristic little French accent still rings in my ear. He had a beautiful wife who, in her pale-blue dress, was the Queen of the Congress in Toulouse.

We enjoyed our new freedom, holidaying in many different places. These holidays were usually connected with scientific Congresses. After the initial humiliation of having failed my basic examinations in England, I made up for lost time. I lectured about my research, my medical and oral surgical experiences. Among many different subjects much emphasis was put about my pioneering work in the prevention of oral cancer.

My lecture in London, in 1962, at the Congress of the International Association of Oral Surgeons, was held in the Festival Hall and the dinner which followed was in the majestic Guildhall. This was followed by many trips: Belluno, Venice, Milan, Siena, Varese, Florence and Porto Venere. In 1966 I went to Paris with Anuci - we always travelled together. From Paris we travelled to Rome where we looked at everything we had the time and chance to. The Villa Borghese was my favourite place. I could hardly wait for the guard to leave the room for a second, so that I could fondle the marble breast of Pauline, the sister of Napoleon in Canova's sculpture. The pillow which she rested upon looked like a real padded quilt and I always stroked it as well. From Rome we sailed to Sardinia where, after the Congress the banquet was in a seaside holiday villa some kilometres from Cagliari, Sardinia's capital. At night, when we returned home, police cars equipped with radios watched the route, because, at that time, the danger of attack by bandits still existed. Anuci and I spent two wonderful weeks in the same villa, Capo Boi, at the seaside. The owner even took me out in her rowing boat and taught me how to fish. Not a single fish took my hook - I think they felt that I was a beginner.

In 1967 I received an invitation to deliver a lecture in Knoxville, USA, in the area of Smokey Mountains, near New Orleans. The temperature was above 100°F. From there we went to New York to meet our dearest old friends, Paul Flesh and Arpad Bernath. In 1970 I lectured again in New York, Brooklyn, and then we made use of our air tickets and flew from New York to Montreal to visit Gabi, my brother-in-law Frici's son. Gabi met us at the airport and it was a lovely reunion. We went to the Espresso Pam-Pam, the meeting place for immigrant Hungarians. I also visited my Dental Surgeon colleague Dr I.H. who had been the Head of a Military Dental Polyclinic in Budapest and was now working from a simple room - as far as I knew unofficially - because he had not by then finished the necessary examinations. From Montreal we flew to Boston where we visited Harvard University. In the vast library there we asked if they had any copies of the scientific works of the Frankl family, and a few minutes later a miniature train loaded with my brother Jozsi's book about Penicillin stopped in front of us. We also met with our famous physicist friend, L. Tisza, who I had taught to throw the javelin, all those years ago. In Boston Mr H., the father of Andrew's first love, collected us in his enormous Cadillac and drove us to Maine and his home. His son-in-law was very rich and owned a specialised fishing fleet with factory and processing ships.

Back in Europe we visited Madrid in Spain. We went to see Franco's mausoleum, a marble palace built underground, with gigantic halls with walls covered with tapestries of unbelievable beauty. It is the resting place of the soldiers of the Spanish Civil War. Now both "Right Wing" and "Left Wing" factions are buried together, in peace.

Apart from the "tourist" side, I gave a lecture at a Congress in Madrid. A German professor also delivered a lecture. After he had started, the organizers announced in Spanish and English, that there was no interpreter to translate from German. They repeated this announcement at regular intervals and the audience burst into laughter each time. I felt sad that this scientist's hard work had all been in vain. At the end of his lecture, I stood up and thanked him.

Marbella, Majorca, Malaga in Spain and Cannes and Juan les Pins on the French Riviera were our other favourite places - not to mention Tunisia and Norway. When In Malaga we went over by bus to the same monastery where Chopin's piano still stands. In Paris, in the cemetery of Père Lachaise, I visited his tomb of white marble, which was, and always has been, covered with fresh pink and red flowers.

Once we took a holiday in Davos and went sightseeing in Liechtenstein, Locarno and Zurich. I had bad pains in my back, and so went to visit Dr. D. Vago, a physician and the daughter of a colleague who had been killed by the Germans. Many years ago, in Budapest, Dr. Vago had been my student. One morning while I was sitting in the bath, she had knocked on the door. She wanted to ask me about the date of her examination. I poked my head out from behind the door and asked her: "Are you fond of me?" - "I love you!" was the answer to which I immediately replied: "You have just passed the examination, with distinction!" She had been a most talented pupil!

In Madeira we visited the grave of the last Hungarian King, Carl IV. Anuci had seen his Coronation in Budapest in 1916.

In Rhodes, as we did in every place, we went to the Synagogue and admired the medieval chair used for circumcision. The guardian of the Synagogue ushered us in and showed us the memorial tablet for the 1700 martyrs deported to Auschwitz by the Nazis in 1944. The Germans had suddenly gone into the courtyards of houses and proclaimed that everybody who was Jewish should come out. Those who had done so were then carried away and never returned. Those who had refused to go into the courtyards. escaped. Even this remote little island wasn't spared the hate.

We spent two holidays in Israel - firstly in Natanya, then in Eilat. In the meantime, I delivered lectures in both Tel Aviv and Jerusalem. On our second trip, and just before we got ready to go to the Airport to return to London, Vera 'phoned us from London. She had just heard on the radio that there had been some trouble there. We were informed at the Airport that the previous day there had been a treacherous machine-gun attack by so-called 'red guard' terrorists. We did

144

not see any trace of blood but, when we looked for the nice lady whom we had met on our arrival in Israel, we were told simply "She will not come back anymore".

So, what actually did life consist of for me in the last 30 years in England? Hard, non-stop work in the surgery, writing, publishing and lecturing scientific studies, and happiness in the physical and intellectual development of our good and honest children - who both succeeded in their careers.

Continuous excitement as in Budapest, about whether or not enough patients would turn up, anxiety regarding the rent for the surgery and the flat.

The 'free' life of England, where there is 'freedom of speech', and one can travel and go around freely, but 'post equitem sedet atra cura' - behind the horseman sits dark anxiety - there was always about you: Tax, and you were always taxed, and for everything. This was difficult to endure and the perpetual worry did not help to raise family spirits. In the end, though, we always earned enough for everything.

Anuci provided the anchor, the strength of the family. She kept the family together with her optimism, with her personality and, with her eternal smile, she settled all the differences, conquered every obstacle, even though at times it must have been very difficult for her. She never hated or held a grudge against anybody, but loved, and was loved by them and she adored her new country.

In the beginning she taught anatomy in a cosmetic institute and, after this, worked as a physiotherapist in a private clinic. Later, however, her state of health interfered with our life. Her heart started to trouble her. She used to help me in the surgery, even with major interventions. Now when she is unable to help, her mere presence gives me strength. Every slope or stair is difficult, if not impossible, and she finds this "restricted" life very painful to bear having been such an active and energetic woman, with such a craving for life. Slowly, but surely she got accustomed to a quiet and more tranquil life.

The dreams haunted me always. After the deportation I dreamt, as everybody else, of hell. We wriggled and struggled, waiting to be executed or worse, and then, seconds before the execution, we woke up sweating, broken, and shattered. After we emigrated to England, the dreams returned again, with the same cruelty and ferocity. They were, by and large, similar. I was trying to leave Hungary and, at the last minute, they refused me permission; that was followed by the well-known awakening with all its sweaty shuddering.

I did not dare to visit Hungary for 28 years, although my son kept trying to persuade me, repeating that nothing evil would happen to me, that things were different now and that everyone would like me. I was still scared, I could not get rid of the thought of the hatred which had accumulated and settled in the Hungarian soul for so many centuries. Where jealousy and envy were the dominant factors of life, where, as a Hungarian poet had said: "Brothers are denouncing brothers".

But in the spring of 1985 my son took me with him on a trip to Budapest. We stayed in the elegant Forum Hotel on the banks of the Danube and, despite my son's worries about me, all of my problems slowly melted away. Instead of bitterness, fear and hatred, I was surrounded by warmth and love. I did not recognise the City - they were building everywhere and I became a little dazed by it all. The affection from members of my family and old friends was really moving, and no one had stopped me at the border. Some months later I returned, this time with my wife. We went to Mátrafured for a two-week holiday, and then on to the Grand Hotel on Margaret Island in Budapest, a favourite place which I used to visit every Saturday after surgery hours. Mátrafured was lovely with its comforting calmness and simplicity, and we felt entirely at home as soon as we got to the Hotel Avar. The espresso was good and the little girls took care of us.

However, during our stay there was a short, but very disturbing moment. In the village of Mátrafured there was a small booth for rifle-practice which I liked to use, and I usually hit the bull's eye. One morning a man, about sixty, came to the booth. He was staggering, visibly drunk, and asked for a rifle. He challenged me to a contest. He was shaky and his shots went all over the place. When he gave the rifle back and was turning away, stabbing his finger in the air, he said, thinking aloud as it were, "Those were beautiful times, when we shot them, one after the other, in the back of the head ..." I was almost paralysed at first and then I shouted at him that that had been the most murderous, bloody period in the history of the world. The booth attendant backed me up, shouting that villains like him should be executed. The man meanwhile, tottered away.

The dark shadow had just for a moment clouded my new happiness. The sound of that "*Whirlwind*" came suddenly close again.

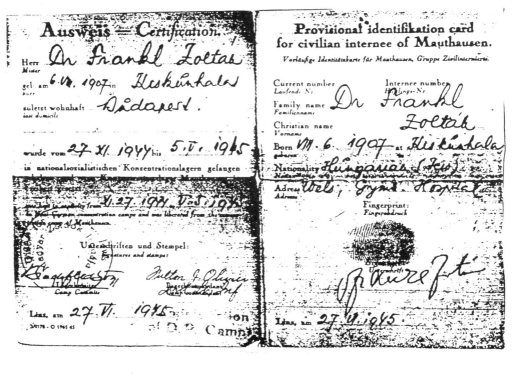

Ausweis — Certification.

Herr / *Mister* Dr Frankl Zoltan

geb. am / *born* 6.VII. 1907 in / *at* Kiskunhalas

zuletzt wohnhaft / *last domicile* Budapest.

wurde vom 27.XI. 1944 bis 5.V. 1945

in nationalsozialistischen Konzentrationslagern gefangen [illegible] Konzentrationslager Mauthausen [illegible]

[illegible] in captivity from XI.27.1944 to V.5.1945

in Nazi German concentration camps and was liberated from the [illegible] camp of Mauthausen

Unterschriften und Stempel: / *Signatures and stamps*

[signature] Lagerkomitee / Camp Committee — Milton J. Olivier, Lagerkommandant / Camp commandant

Linz, am 27.VI. 1945 [illegible] on [illegible] of D.P. Camp

3/0178 - O 1965 45

Provisional identifikation card for civilian internee of Mauthausen.

Vorläufige Identitätskarte für Mauthausen, Gruppe Zivilinternierte.

Current number / *Laufende Nr.* — Internee number / *Häftlings-Nr.*

Family name / *Familienname* Dr Frankl

Christian name / *Vorname* Zoltán

Born / *geboren* VII. 6. 1907 at Kiskunhalas

Nationality / *Nationalität* Hungarian (Jew)

Adress / *Adresse* Wels, Gymn. Hospital

Fingerprint: / *Fingerabdruck*

Unterschrift [signature]

Linz, am 27.VI.1945.

MILITARY GOVERNMENT
OF GERMANY

MILITÄRREGIERUNG-BEFREIUNG — **B** 740662
MILITARY GOVERNMENT EXEMPTION

Datum der Ausstellung / *Date Issued* 25 June 45 — Wird unwirksam am / *Expires on* 1 Aug 45

Name / *Name* Dr. Z. Frankl

Anschrift / *Address* Dr. Schauerstr. 9 — Wohnort / *Town* Wels

Ausweiskarte Klasse / *Identity Card Type* — Nr. / *No.*

Unterschrift des Inhabers / *Signature of Holder* [signature]

ANWEISUNGEN: Diese Befreiung ist im Namen des Militärregierung ausgestellt worden. Sie ist nicht übertragbar, darf nicht abgeändert oder vernichtet werden und ist nur gültig in Verbindung mit der Ausweiskarte des Inhabers. Der Verlust dieser Karte muss der Polizei gemeldet werden. Gefundene oder unwirksam gewordene Karten müssen an die ausstellende Behörde zurückgegeben werden.

INSTRUCTIONS: This exemption is issued by Military Government. It is not transferable, must not be altered or destroyed, and is only valid when used in conjunction with the holder's identity card. The loss of this card must be reported to the police. If found, or on expiration of validity, this card must be returned to the issuing authority.